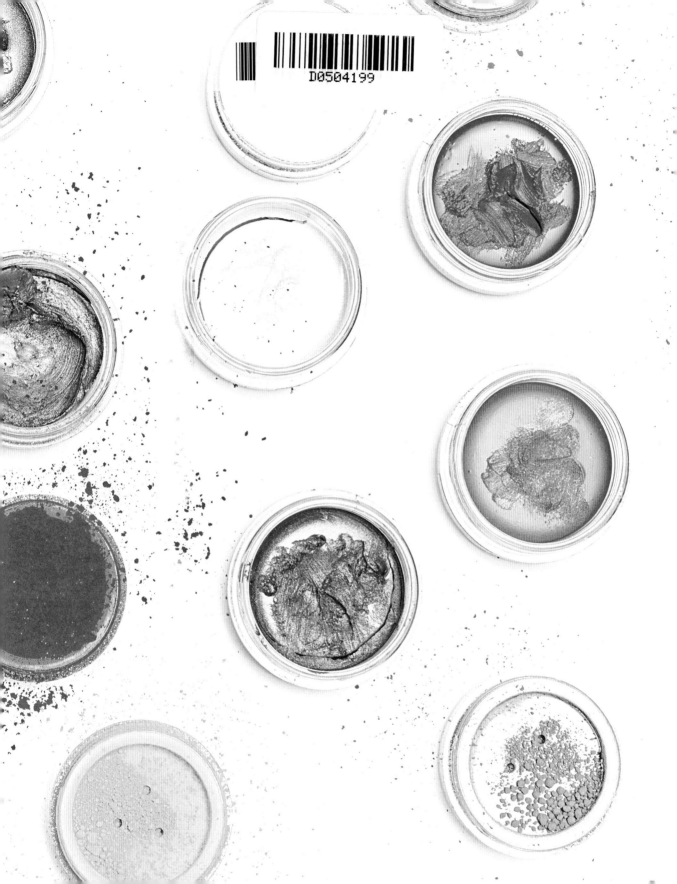

D0504199

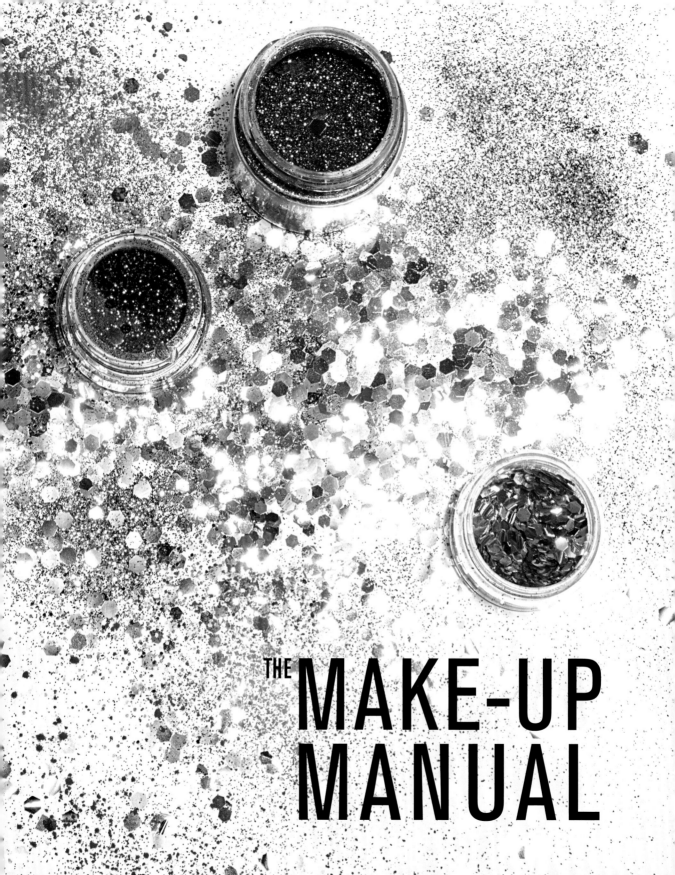

THE MAKE-UP MANUAL

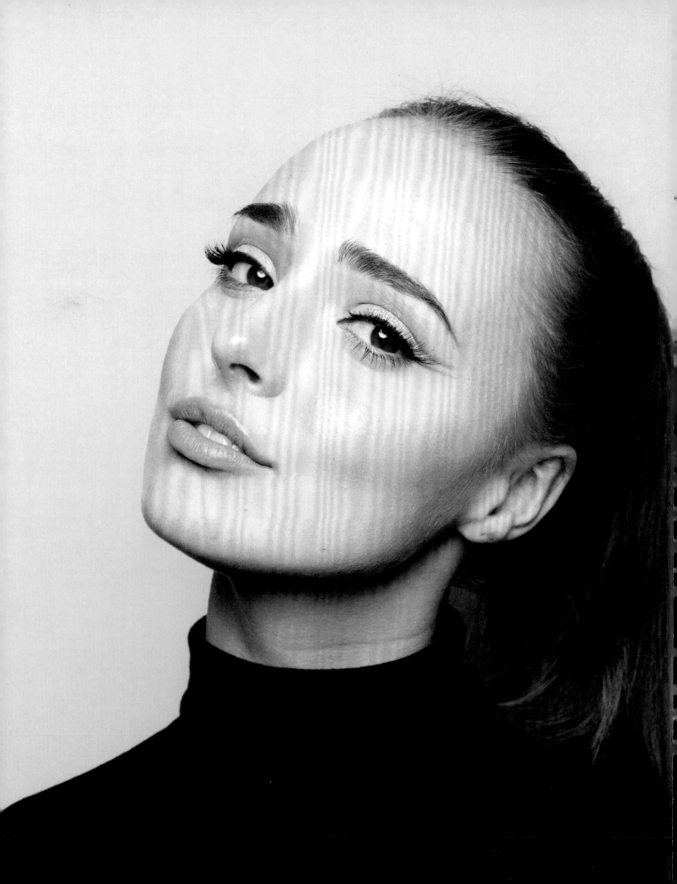

THE MAKE-UP MANUAL

Your beauty guide for brows, eyes, skin, lips and more

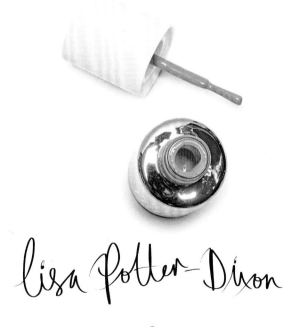

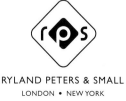

Lisa Potter-Dixon

rps

RYLAND PETERS & SMALL
LONDON • NEW YORK

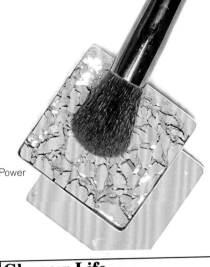

Designer Barbara Zuñiga
Commissioning editor Stephanie Milner
Production Mai-Ling Collyer
Art director Leslie Harrington
Editorial director Julia Charles
Publisher Cindy Richards

Photographer Rhys Frampton
Make-up artist Lisa Potter-Dixon
Make-up assistants Lauren Hogsden and Laurretta Power
Hair stylist Mathieu Clabaux
Illustrator Sally Faye Cotterill
Indexer Vanessa Bird

First published in 2017 by
Ryland Peters & Small
20–21 Jockey's Fields, London WC1R 4BW
and
341 E 116th St, New York NY 10029
www.rylandpeters.com

10 9 8 7 6 5 4 3 2 1

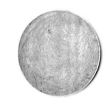

ISBN: 978-1-84975-804-8

Printed in China

Disclaimer:
The views expressed in this book are those of the author but they
are general views only and readers are urged to consult a relevant
and qualified specialist or physician for individual advice before
beginning any beauty regimen. This book was not created in
the context of the author's employment with Benefit Cosmetics
and/or any Benefit group company. The views expressed in this
book do not necessarily represent the views of Benefit. Ryland
Peters & Small hereby exclude all liability to the extent permitted
by law for any errors or omissions in this book and for any loss,
damage or expense (whether direct or indirect) suffered by a
third party relying on any information contained in this book.

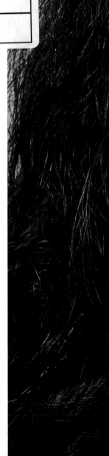

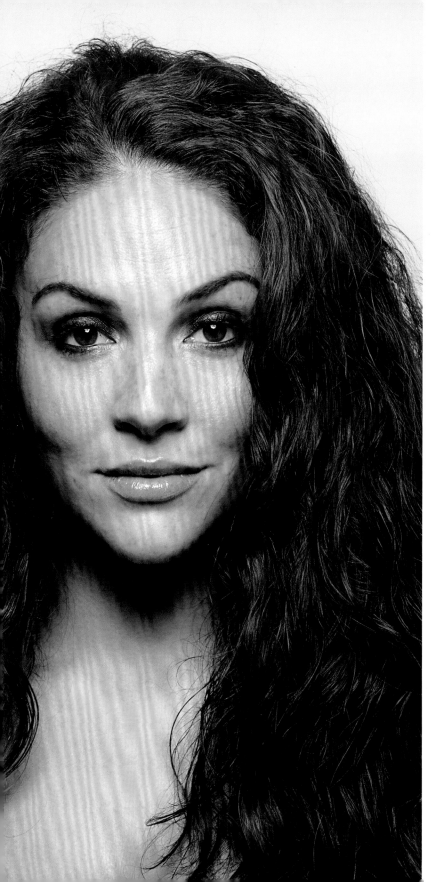

Contents

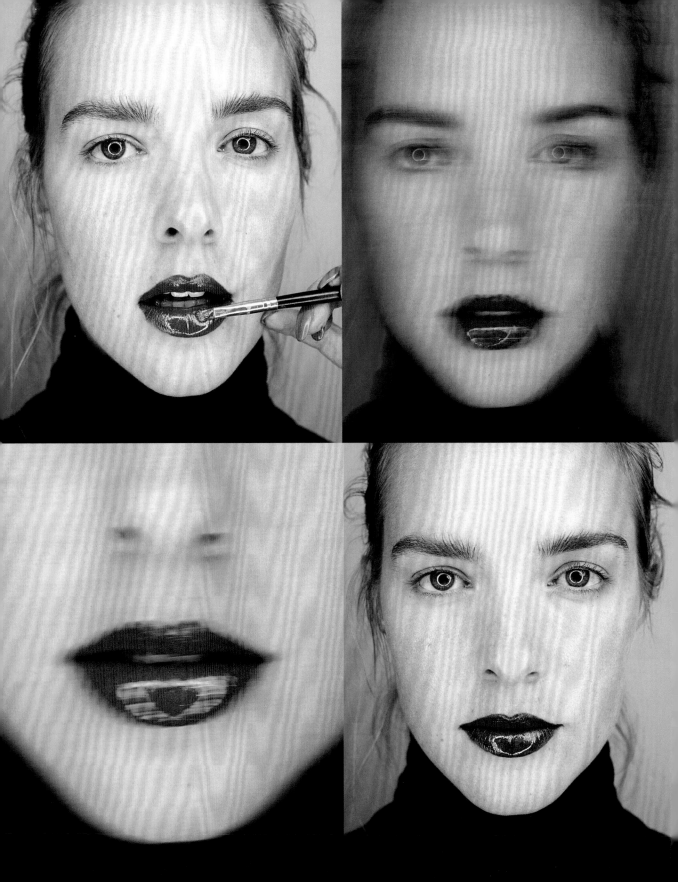

Foreword

by Sophie Beresiner, Beauty Director, ELLE UK

Having worked closely with Lisa Potter-Dixon for almost a decade I've had the pleasure of watching her career and her craft evolve into something entirely unique. I call her a 'user-friendly' make-up artist. It is impossible not to warm to her effusive charm. She generates the most amazing ideas and she is so easy to learn from.

This book is an informative marvel, a visual feast, a guide book to looking like the best version of you and essentially becoming your own make-up artist. It's also a little peek into the crazy, cool and always creative life of Lisa.

I'm always impressed by Lisa's work and her ability to make everyone, from the most hardened make-up-phobes to those stuck in old habits, to try new things, embrace their beauty and enjoy wearing the latest looks. As the leader of the Power Brow Revolution, she has taught me exactly how important my own eyebrows are, so much so that I refuse to let anyone else touch them!

Lisa is the kind of approachable, make-up artist you want to be your friend – not least because she can make you look completely fantastic at the drop of a hat. Lucky for me, she has become just that, and seeing her genius and personality laid out over the following pages means that you get to benefit too.

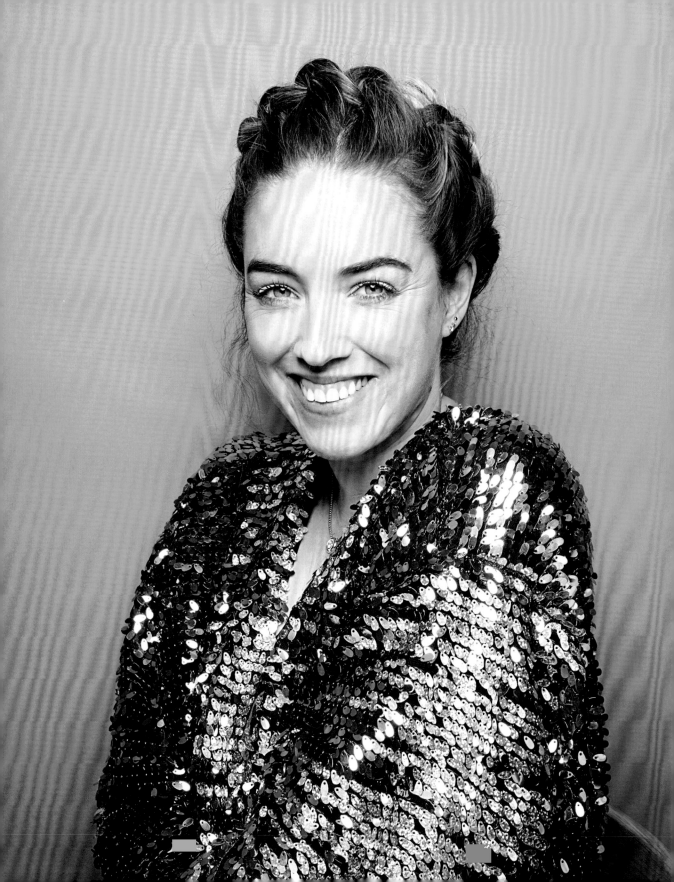

Hi guys,

Welcome to your make-up manual. This book is filled with knowledge from my 12 years of experience as a make-up artist. My job has taken me around the globe and I've worked on some beautiful faces over the years, creating gorgeous and, sometimes, slightly crazy make-up looks. However, the thing I love most about make-up is how it makes you feel. With a touch of concealer or a swipe of a lipstick, you can instantly feel better, happier and more confident.

You do not need to be a make-up artist to be good at applying it. But, because hundreds if not thousands of women have told me, I know that a lot of women still find it a challenge. So I'm here to change all of that. Make-up is not something to be feared – remember, you can always take it off.

In this manual you'll find a comprehensive guide that leads you through skincare routines, beauty dilemmas, the power of the brow, flawless skin, luscious lips and a number of gorgeous make-up looks, with a few glittery ones thrown in there too!

So learn, play, experiment and create. And always remember that you are beautiful with or without make up, but a little bit of red lipstick never hurt anyone! Tag me in your creations @Lisa_Benefit and #LearnWithLisa – I love to see how gorgeous you all are!

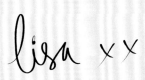 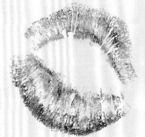

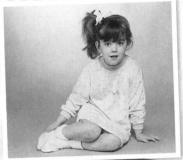

My mum tried to pass on her modelling gene – it didn't work out...

About me

I've loved make-up ever since I can remember. I used to save up my pocket money to buy products to use on my Girl's World head toy. Although most of it would end up on my little sisters' faces (and occasionally on my brother's), much to their despair!

In my early teens, I was a competitive disco dancer. I could never master the splits as well as I could the sequins. And I think this is where my love of all things sparkly came into play. I literally used to stick sequins all over my face for dance competitions!

At school in the 1990s, 'heather shimmer' lipstick (remember that awful, purply brown, shimmery shade!) was my everything. I wouldn't leave my house without that and my cherry red Dr. Martens™ boots! I'd practise my make-up skills on my friends for school discos, nominate myself to paint the faces of everyone acting in school plays and I'd continue to harass my sisters with glitter and lip gloss. All of this continued through college and university, and, although my love for make-up was obvious, I didn't really consider that it could become my full-time job until I joined Benefit.

This is when my make-up world lit up! As well as managing the Covent Garden boutique, I used to run events and masterclasses at any opportunity. Offering my skills to local journalists who, at the time, had absolutely no idea who I was, but who, for some reason, started to let me make up their faces and wax their brows for all sorts of special occasions. This started to open doors into the fashion industry. I took every opportunity I could see, as well as continuing to run the successful Benefit boutique.

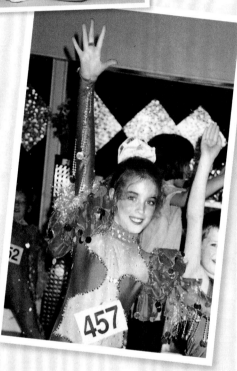

Where my love of sequins and glitter began

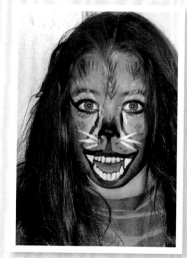

A classic make-up look from my amateur theatre days!

Me and my dog, Snoopy

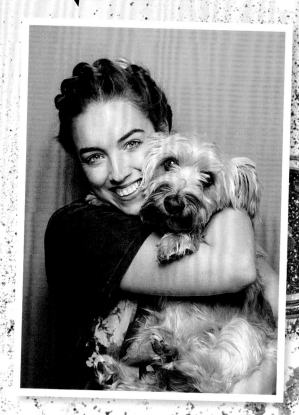

Asking the Benefit UK team to become their first ever Head Make-up Artist and Brow Artist, was one of the most nerve-racking days ever. However, in the typical Benefit way, I was not only given this opportunity, but I was supported 100 per cent by the entire team. This support continues today and it is has made me want to become the best that I can possibly be.

Since then and over the past five years, I have worked tirelessly to learn and develop as a make-up artist. I now regularly shoot with magazines and fashion designers, travelling the globe and working on some of the most beautiful faces in the world. I head up shows at London Fashion Week and host beauty slots on numerous TV shows, as well as having my own Youtube channel, where I share yet more of my insider secrets. I now have an incredible team that just keeps on growing. Some people look at me and say, 'Wow, you've got the dream job!' My answer is always, 'Yes, I have, but I've worked for it – that's for sure!'

And here I am, writing my second book! The 1997 heather-shimmer-wearing Lisa could never have dreamt of this. And it really has only been possible because of the support I've had from my amazing husband, friends, family and colleagues. They've always believed in me and I've (nearly) always believed in myself.

Just remember, you can achieve whatever you want to achieve. It just takes hard work, persistence, passion and a touch of sparkle.

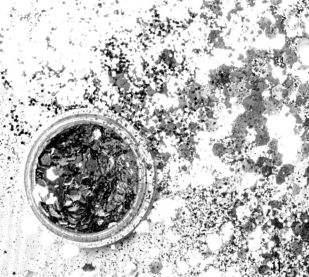

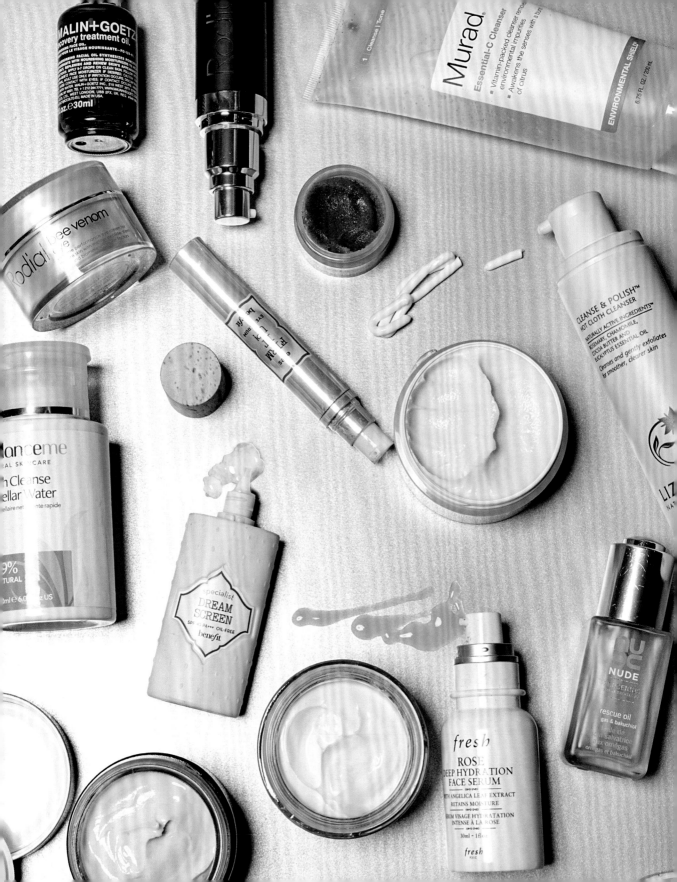

Skin secrets

I've been obsessed with skincare since I was about 12 years old. I have never slept in my make-up and have been known to remove my friends' make-up for them when they have fallen asleep after a night out!

There are a variety of skin types out there. Sometimes our skin type stays the same forever, sometimes it adjusts depending on the season, time of the month, illness, age, pregnancy – there are countless things that can affect our skin.

I am not a facialist or a skincare specialist, but having worked with thousands of different women over the years, all with different dilemmas, and having listened to and read advice from skin experts such as Caroline Hirons, Liz Earle, Mandy Oxley-Swan and Alison Young; I certainly know a thing or two.

So within these pages are the basic skincare rules that I follow. Here's to beautiful, glowing skin!

Types of skin

Not knowing what skin type you have can be frustrating as it means you're probably not picking the right skincare products. Here's a quick breakdown of the most common skin types to give you a helping hand, as well as my top product for each type. See page 23 for more of my top products.

Normal

You have this skin type if...

* You wouldn't describe your skin as oily or dry; it just looks and feels even ('normal') in all areas
* Any oiliness or dryness you do experience is rare
* Your pores are not enlarged or visible
* You rarely/never feel you need to touch up your powder during the day
* Your skin doesn't feel tight or dry at the end of the day, nor is it obviously shiny
* Your skin tone is fairly even, with no brown or red spots or patches

Top product: Fresh Soy Face Cleanser

Oily

You have this skin type if...

* You have enlarged pores
* Your complexion is always/often too shiny
* You always/often have blackheads, pimples or other blemishes
* Your make-up doesn't stay in place for long

Top product: Liz Earle Super Skin Facial Oil

Dry

You have this skin type if...

* You have almost invisible pores
* Your complexion is dull and rough
* You sometimes/always get red patches
* Your skin isn't very elastic
* You have visible lines

Top product: Benefit Total Moisturise Facial Cream

Combination

You have this skin type if...

* Your pores look larger than normal, because they are more open
* You have blackheads
* Your skin is shiny
* You have dry areas

Top product: Liz Earle Cleanse and Polish

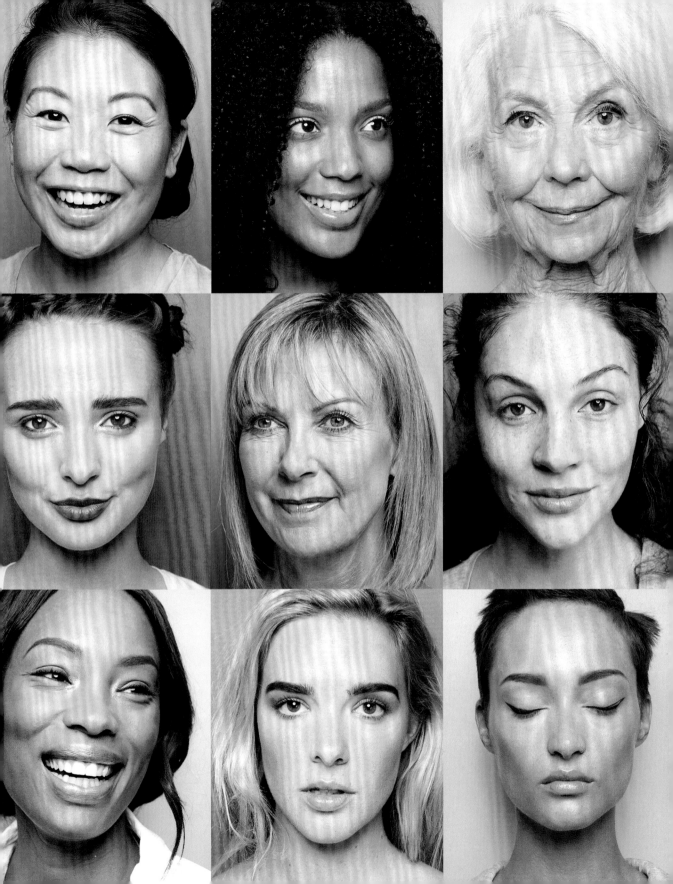

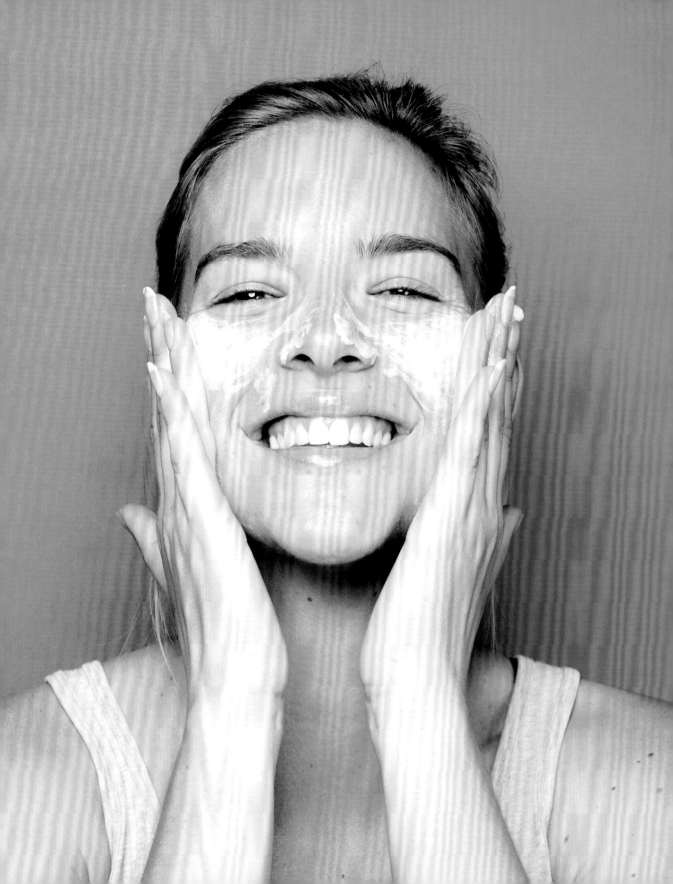

The beauty regime

Whether you wear make-up or not, a skincare routine is essential. Your skin is precious and the more you look after it, the better you'll look and feel. These are my basic steps that I believe you should follow twice a day, morning and night, whatever your age, whatever your skin type. (Remember, it's never too late to start taking care of your skin.)

Step 1

Double cleanse your face. Cleansing once removes make-up and grime. Cleansing twice deep cleans your face. I love a cream cleanser for this process as they tend to remove all make-up, including anything waterproof. Apply the cream with clean fingers and remove with a flannel or a face cloth. If you haven't used one of these before, then give it a go! You'll literally see the daily grime lift off with the cream – sounds gross, right?! Well, it is a bit, but a flannel or face cloth will show you what you're taking off, and when you've double cleansed you should be able to see that there's nothing left on your skin.

NOTE: Avoid face wipes unless it is an absolute beauty emergency (i.e. you're in a muddy field at a festival with no access to running water) as these dry your skin out and basically do, well, nothing!

Top tip

Splash your face with (as cold as possible) cold water after you've cleansed it to close pores and tighten skin.

Step 2

Now for serum. Serums are the secret weapons of the skincare world. These beauties penetrate the skin quickly to give your skin all the goodness it needs. Make sure you pick a serum that's right for your skin type (see pages 14–15). These are powerful little things so you don't want to be applying the wrong type. Massage the serum into your face and neck.

Step 3 (optional)

Apply facial oil. I'm obsessed with facial oil. I love oils as they are packed full of vitamins and omega fats that work hard to hydrate your skin beautifully. This is an optional step but if you haven't used a facial oil before then give it a go. I apply mine morning and night but for first-timers, try it at night to start with.

Step 4

Moisturize after serum or oil. My moisturizer is the product I change the most, mainly because there are so many out there and I get drawn in by beautiful packaging. I use a day cream in the morning as they tend to be more lightweight, meaning I can apply my make-up straight over the top. And a night cream at night as these are richer and your skin works harder at night. Moisturizers keep your skin hydrated and looking plump.

Step 5

Finish off with an eye cream. A lot of people think the benefits of eye creams are a myth. My theory is that your eye area needs an extra boost (just like when you use concealer under eyes). The skin around the eye is the thinnest area on your face. There are tonnes of eye creams out there. Pick one that suits your dilemma. Whether that be dark circles, ageing or puffiness. Pat it around the orbital bone. (That's the bone you can feel all the way around your eye. It leads to your brow bone.) Blend upwards towards the eye using your ring finger as this has the softest touch.

And there you have it: a restorative beauty regime that can be performed in under 5 minutes. If you ask me it's always worth taking the time to take care of your skin.

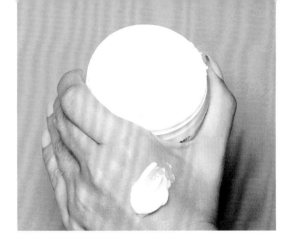

Beauty extras

As well as the twice-daily beauty regime on page 17, everyone should...

Exfoliate

Exfoliating is wonderful for your skin. It removes dead cells and brightens up the skin beneath. Exfoliate after cleansing (see Step 1, page 17) twice a week, by massaging exfoliator into your skin, then washing off.

Apply SPF

SPF creams are so important as they protect from the sun's harmful UV rays. Most moisturizers now include an SPF, however, I still apply an SPF cream before moisturizer every morning, usually SPF 45.

Use lip balm

I apply lip balm every night as my lips dry out very easily. As a result, I don't use as much in the day as I find that the more you use a lip balm, the less it actually works.

Use face masks

I love face masks. These always feel like a treat. I usually apply these once a week, on a Sunday.

Acne stations

My husband and sisters have all suffered with severe acne at different times. It's such a frustrating problem that can really knock your confidence. It is caused by many different things, from hormone and stress levels to diet and a low immune system.

Later in this book, I talk about the best way to cover up blemishes with make-up, but ultimately, there's no magic solution. However, skincare is vital to the healing and prevention of spots.

So when it comes to acne and skincare this is what I recommend:

✱ Never burst a blemish if it's red! Red equals STOP! You'll make it angry. It's fine to get rid of white heads after a bath or shower as long as you do it gently!

✱ Avoid soaps and foaming washes. These will irritate acne-prone skin.

✱ Stay away from anything that has alcohol as its main ingredient (unless it's a piña colada!) These products can cause you a lot of pain when applied to problem areas and they can dry the skin out too much.

✱ DON'T avoid facial oils and moisturizers. So many people with acne think that their skin doesn't need these, or that it's going to make your skin worse. It is in fact the complete opposite. As long as you stick to light, plant-derived facial oils, such as Artemis Hydroactive Cellular Face Oil, your skin will thank you for it. These oils can help to reduce inflammation and redness.

✱ Avoid heavy moisturizers with shea butter content as this can clog the pores.

✱ If I have an awful spot, one of those volcano-like ones, I smear a bit of manuka honey on it. Manuka is packed full of goodness and I find this helps to take the inflammation down.

Body beauty

Okay, so now your face is gorgeous and clean, but don't forget your body. You need to look after this just as much.

Exfoliate

I use a body brush every day just before bathing as this helps to encourage good circulation, removes dead skin cells and helps combat cellulite. I also love a body exfoliator. Especially one that includes soothing oils. They make your skin feel incredible. Apply body exfoliator in a circular motion all over the skin and wash off.

Apply bath oils

Bath oils are a quick way to relax and moisturize the skin (although I still always moisturize, too). They tend to include aromatherapy oils which smell incredible and help you to relax. Put a few drops in your bath and enjoy!

Use body moisturizer

I moisturize my body every evening. It keeps your skin feeling supple and looking glowing. Really focus on your legs and elbows as these tend to get extra dry.

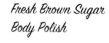

Fresh Brown Sugar Body Polish

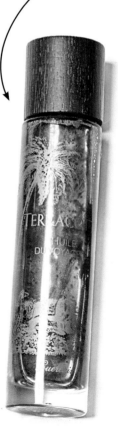

Guerlain Terracotta Huile du Voyageur Nourishing Dry Oil

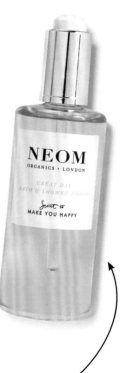

Neom Organics Perfect Night's Sleep Bath & Shower Drops

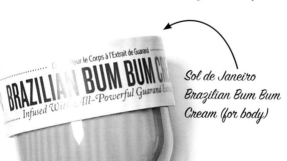

Sol de Janeiro Brazilian Bum Bum Cream (for body)

Homemade face masks

I love a good face mask. Combine it with a bubble bath and RELAX! There are so many great ready-made masks out there, but I enjoy making my own. Mainly because I then know exactly what is in them. We all have different skin issues, so I've listed my favourite recipes for easing various dilemmas.

For a perfect glow

Everyone wants glowing skin. And yes, you can add highlighter to your heart's content. But a natural, healthy glow starts with naked skin. You'll find you need to wear less make-up if your skin is in good condition. These are two of my favourite homemade face masks, perfect before (or after) a big night out!

The first of two masks for the perfect glow contains coffee, which isn't just good for your soul; it's also good for your skin. Applied topically, coffee helps to reduce

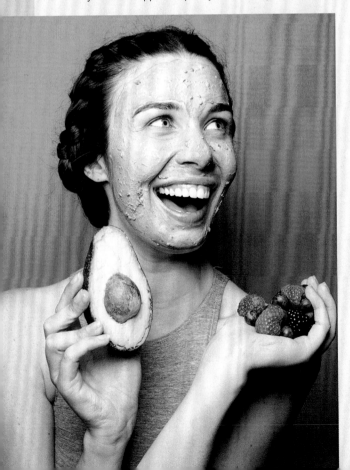

inflammation, redness and the appearance of dark circles. The cocoa powder in this mask is a good source of antioxidants, which repair skin damage, and contains high levels of sulphur, which is great for fighting acne. But before you chuck your caramel latte over your face, read the recipe below.

The second mask is amazing for brightening your skin. But it also tastes delicious. I've been known to double the recipe just so I have some to eat while I wait!

The 'everything is better with coffee' mask

4 tablespoons ground organic coffee beans
2 tablespoons unsweetened cocoa powder
3 tablespoons almond milk
1 tablespoon freshly squeezed lemon juice
1 tablespoon honey

Rinse your face with water and pat dry. Mix all the ingredients together and apply the mixture directly to the skin of your face. Leave for 20 minutes, then rinse off with cool water.

The 'good luck trying not to eat it' mask

½ banana
½ avocado
6 blueberries
1 tablespoon freshly squeezed orange juice
1 tablespoon honey

Rinse your face with water and pat dry. Mash the banana, avocado and blueberries together, then mix in the orange juice and honey. Apply to the face and keep the mixture on for 15 minutes. Rinse with lukewarm water, then moisturize.

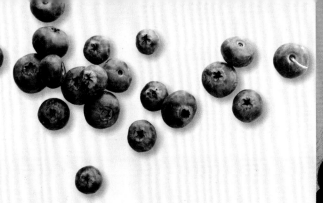

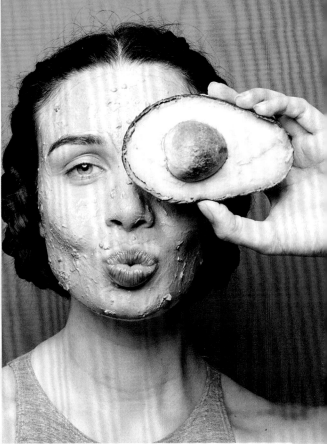

For acne

Acne and spots are infuriating. Whether you get that one volcano the same day as a huge presentation, or you feel like a boxer in a never-ending fight with spots, pimples, whatever you want to call them, acne has been the bane of all of our lives at some point. Looking after your skin is vital and this face mask includes two of the more powerful treatments for combating spots. Cinnamon and honey both have anti-microbial and anti-inflammatory properties, meaning that they can help reduce blemishes naturally. Try this mask twice a week for a month. Take a before and after picture to see if your skin has improved.

The 'it's time to fight back' mask

2 tablespoons honey (preferably manuka honey for its
   health-giving properties)
1 teaspoon ground cinnamon

Rinse your face with water and pat dry. Mix the honey and cinnamon together until they are thoroughly blended and have formed a sort of paste. Apply the mixture directly to your face (or trouble area) and leave on for 10–15 minutes. Rinse off completely, and pat your face dry.

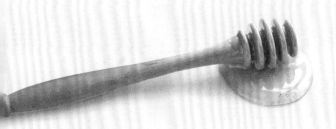

For dry skin

I suffer with dry skin on my face and hands. This mask has been a saviour for me. Coconut oil and avocado are packed with natural essential oils that nourish the skin wonderfully. Try this mask twice a week and watch that dry skin vanish.

The 'dry skin be gone' mask

2 tablespoons coconut oil, plus extra to moisturize
½ avocado
3 drops frankincense essential oil

Mix the coconut oil with the avocado. Both are full of essential oils perfect to nourish dry skin. Add the frankincense essential oil – this is great for cellular regeneration. Apply to the face and keep the mixture on for 20 minutes, then rinse off, pat dry and add a layer of coconut oil to moisturize.

Age

As we get older, our skin changes. I like to think that the more wrinkles you have, the better the life you have lived. And those fine lines around your eyes, well, the more of those you have, the more you've laughed. And laughter is good for the soul.

There's no magic elixir to totally stop wrinkles forming or halt the ageing process (yet!) There are obviously multiple surgical procedures you can have and I definitely understand why women have botox treatments and face-lifts, but I haven't delved into that side of anti-ageing treatment yet, and I'm not sure if it's something that I ever will do. But never say never, hey?! Instead, I advocate looking after your skin. Protect it with SPF creams, always remove your make-up at night and invest in good-quality skincare products.

Our skin gets thinner as we get older and we start to lose the elasticity and plumpness of the surface, especially in the face. But if you treat your skin with love and respect, you will, without doubt, slow down the ageing process. So, instead of buying that pair of shoes this month, buy that moisturizer.

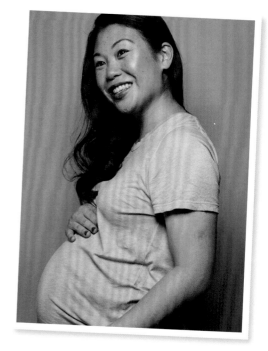

Pregnancy

Your body changes a lot during pregnancy, and this can affect your skin. Here are a few things to watch out for and change in your skincare routine during pregnancy.

Firstly, does the 'pregnancy glow' really exist? Yes, is the answer! Your skin retains moisture during pregnancy which plumps it up and gives that magical glow. Yay! However, with pregnancy comes hormones and lots of them. Increased levels of hormones can cause increased production of oil, meaning that you are more prone to spots, clogged pores and blemishes; and you can start to see pigmentation marks appear or freckles darken.

So just be prepared to change your skincare routine during pregnancy – you may not need to stick with the routine after pregnancy but refer to the Types of Skin chart on page 14 to understand how your skin is changing.

Any don't forget to oil that bump – Bio-Oil™ and coconut oil keep skin moisturized and stave off stretch marks and scarring. Apply an oil to your body and bump daily.

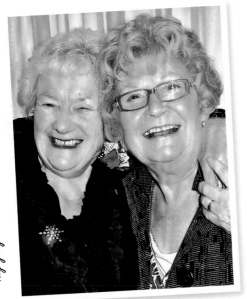

My gorgeous Nans!

My favourite skincare products

Cleansers

Cetaphil Gentle Skin Cleanser (save) This fragrance-free cleanser removes dirt without stripping the skin's natural oils or disturbing its pH balance.

Fresh Soy Face Cleanser (spend) This is my daily cleanser. It's full of amino-acid-rich soy proteins as well as rose water and cucumber to soothe the skin.

Liz Earle Cleanse and Polish (spend) This iconic cleanser is enriched with cocoa butter to soften, smooth and moisturise, and rosemary chamomile and eucalyptus to tone, soothe and purify. Great for removing make-up.

EVE LOM Cleanser (splurge) This easily removes waterproof make-up and contains antiseptic clove oil, eucalyptus oil which drain toxins, toning hops oil and Egyptian chamomile and cocoa butter which softens skin.

Moisturizers

Nivea Crème (save) An iconic moisturizer which is said to share 30 ingredients with CRÈME DE LA MER (see Eye Creams) for a tenth of the price.

Benefit Total Moisture Facial Cream (spend) Containing mango butter, a plant-based emollient, I use this rich moisturizing cream at night all year round.

Fresh Black Tea Age-delay Cream (splurge) Containing antioxidant black tea and anti-ageing lychee seed and blackberry leaf extracts and polysaccharides.

Facial oils

Coconut oil (save) This natural oil is anti-bacterial, anti-fungal and moisturizing for face, body, hair and nails!

Sanctuary Spa Therapist's Secret Facial Oil (save) The combination of sunflower, wheatgerm, jojoba and rosehip oils revives tired, dull, lacklustre skin.

Balance Me Radiance Face Oil (spend) Reduces scarring, redness and pigmentation thanks to the Amazonian buriti nut, camellia and rosehip oils.

Serums

Nip+Fab Dragon's Blood Fix Plumping Serum (save) Amazing for hydrating skin thanks to the hyaluronic acid, velvet flower and dragon blood.

ELEMIS Pro-Collagen Super Serum Elixir (spend) This is a super-concentrated, anti-ageing serum which is powered by the unique blend of tri-peptides, African birch bark, red seaweed and padina pavonica. Hyaluronic acid, combined with omega-rich camelina oil provides superior moisturization too.

Rodial Snake Serum O2 (splurge) I love Rodial and am obsessed with their snake collection. The snake-venom-inspired peptide reduces mimic wrinkles (caused by facial movement) and smoothes skin.

Eye creams

Benefit It's Potent! Eye Cream (spend) The go-to eye cream that reduces dark circles.

CRÈME DE LA MER The Eye Concentrate (splurge) This iconic eye cream is incredible for visibly diminishing dark circles thanks to the hematite. The metal applicator takes down puffiness too.

Treatments

Murad Intensive-C Radiance Peel (spend) This is an intense treatment, full of glycolic acid that exfoliates skin and accelerates cell turnover. It also includes vitamin C and Indian fig for firm skin.

Perricone MD High Potency Face Firming Activator (splurge) The combination of antioxidant alpha lipoic acid and the cell stabilizer DMAE minimizes the appearance, length, width and depth of wrinkles.

Fresh Crème Ancienne Ultimate Nourishing Honey Mask (splurge) This is a one-of-a-kind hydrating treatment that instantly melts into the skin and leaves it feeling hydrated for hours.

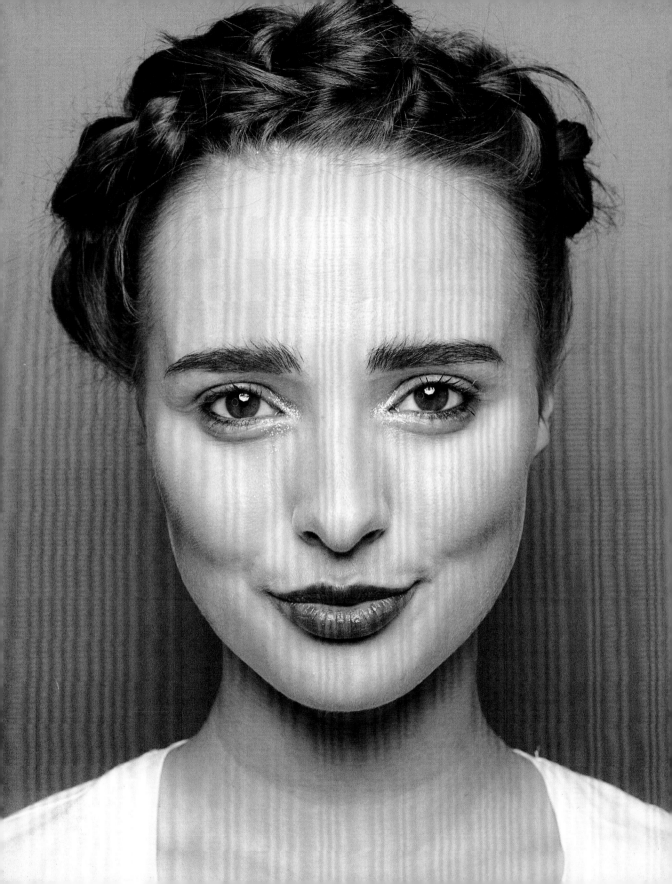

All about the base

Perfecting your base is an important part of creating any make-up look. Some people find they need to cover the whole face with foundation and use concealer and colour correctors, while others will opt for a lighter coverage. You may even choose to vary this for different occasions: weddings and parties tend to require a heavier hand, but you'll need very little during the day, on holiday or if that's just what you prefer.

Over the next few pages, I discuss what foundation you should use and how to use it and help you to understand the different types of concealers available before showing step by step how to eliminate rosacea, dark circles, blemishes and more.

Once you've got the hang of applying your base, there'll be no stopping you from trying all the fabulous looks in this book.

Thank goodness for foundation

Foundation is the make-up product that makes the biggest difference. I rarely go out without some sort of base. Fresh-looking skin is everything! And skin is my thing! I love making a woman look like she has no make-up on (when in fact she has at least four products on).

It's also the one make-up product that so many women get wrong at home. Of course, it's easy to go wrong when there are just *so* many products out there. From liquid to powder, BB to CC cream, how do you know which one's right for you?

Over the next few pages I'll teach you how to pick the right shade and product for you. No more make-up masks or orange tides around the hairline and neck, I promise!

Primer

Let's start at the beginning with primer. This is a relatively new product in the everyday woman's make-up bag. Until recently it was pretty much a make-up artist's secret. As most primers are invisible once on the skin, you may think, 'Why do I need this?' Here's why: a primer gives you an even base ready for foundation. It can minimize the appearance of pores and fine lines, knock back discoloration and keep your make-up in place for longer. All pretty good reasons to use it, hey!

Liquid foundation

The most common foundation and suitable for all skin types, this is my favourite type of base. Opt for an oil-free formula if you have oily skin. They usually give a medium coverage and a dewy finish (unless you opt for a matte product). Liquid foundation blends well whether you use your fingers, a brush or a sponge to apply it. I love using a fluffy eyeshadow brush for blending foundation – see why on page 28.

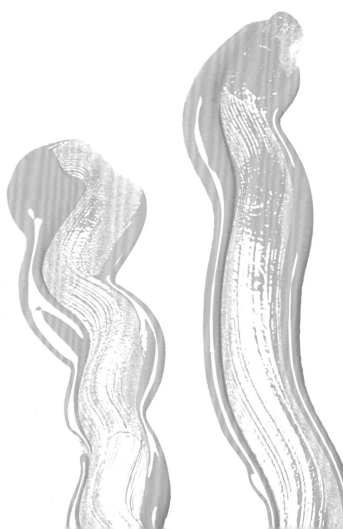

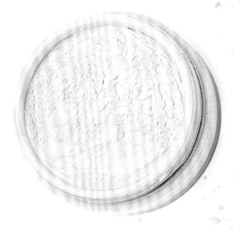

Powder foundation

The right powder is great to take away excess shine. Translucent, lightweight powers are best for that. I'm not a huge fan of full foundation powders because I find that they can cake throughout the day. They can also age you as they tend to sit in fine lines and pores. If you have dry skin, avoid them at all cost. If you have oily skin, don't think that this is your only option. Try an oil-free liquid foundation with a dusting of translucent powder over your T-zone to target the problem area.

Cream foundation

These foundations tend to be heavier than a liquid foundation. They are usually matte, which is great if you have scars on the face and want to avoid excess shine around scarring that you might find are highlighted with liquid foundations. These are great for an evening look due to their stay-put nature.

Tinted moisturizers

This is my favourite holiday base! Tinted moisturizers tend to give a lovely healthy glow with a light coverage. Most have SPF in them (although I recommend using a separate SPF and a separate moisturizer underneath your base). This is the perfect 'chuck it on' product, but don't expect it to give you the coverage of foundation. Do expect it to enhance your skin without looking heavy.

BB (Blemish Balm) and CC (Colour Corrector) creams

I'm not a huge fan of either of these products. I find BB creams are too light (I prefer a tinted moisturizer for a super-light base). And I find that CC creams usually need another product over the top of them because the undertone colour rarely matches a skin tone. They're good if you need to colour correct your skin or if you want a super-light base, but personally, I'd use a tinted moisturizer for these occasions.

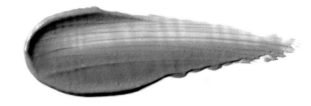

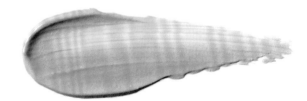

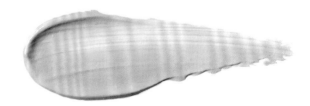

How to apply foundation

Liquid and cream

There are so many different techniques and tools for applying foundation, using brushes, sponges or your fingers. But my favourite technique for liquid and cream foundations is to use something made for your eyes, not your face! And that is a fluffy eyeshadow brush (see pages 60–61). Now this takes a bit more time than using the likes of a sponge or a foundation brush, but it's worth it. Your skin will look flawless and airbrushed and the foundation will stay on for longer. Yay!

step 1 After skincare, apply your preferred primer.

step 2 (optional) This is an LPD special. If you want dewy looking skin, buff a liquid highlighter all over your face using a blusher brush. If you have oily skin you should avoid applying the highlighter on the T-zone and chin.

step 3 Apply colour corrector if needed (see page 31). Dip the fluffy eyeshadow brush into your foundation (I like to use the back of my hand as a palette) and buff it onto the skin in circular motions. Because you're using a small brush, you can build up the product where you need more coverage, and blend it lightly into areas that you don't need as much coverage. You should never just apply one thick layer of foundation but instead target the areas that need coverage the most.

step 4 Add concealer where necessary and finish with a light translucent powder on the T-zone and chin if you tend to be a little shiny. Don't powder the cheeks or nose as these areas look best dewy and fresh.

NOTE: Check out my YouTube video on 'How to get natural, flawless skin' for a tutorial on applying foundation (see page 158).

Powder

Blusher brushes are better than the smaller eyeshadow brushes for powder foundation because they spread the product evenly and quickly without caking.

step 1 Apply primer, colour corrector and concealer as with liquid and cream foundation (left).

step 2 Buff the foundation all over the face using a kabuki brush (see pages 60–61).

Top tip
If your base ever looks too heavy, spritz your skin with a hydrating spray to give it a natural finish without removing any make-up.

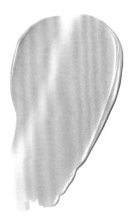
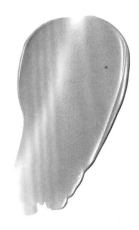

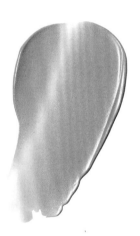

Change with the seasons

As your skin changes through the seasons, you may need to change your foundation shade. I usually have a tinted moisturizer for Summer and a liquid foundation for Spring, Autumn/Fall and Winter. I'm also obsessed with liquid bronzers. These are amazing for warming up your complexion if your foundation seems a bit pale. If your foundation seems a bit dark once your tan fades, try mixing it with your moisturizer to lighten it.

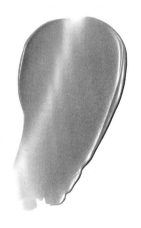

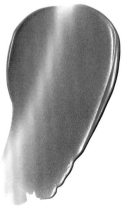
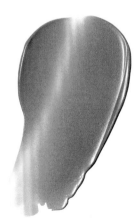

Concealers

I love concealer nearly as much as I love my husband! (Nearly!) They cover a multitude of sins and can look flawless and natural if applied correctly. First things first, which concealer is right for you? Well, it's actually pretty straightforward…

Use a liquid-based concealer under the eyes

for hydrating, preventing creases and brightening the eyes

Use a cream-based concealer on your face

for good coverage, blending with foundation and matching your skin tone

The key to concealing is application. You may have a preference of how you apply yours, but opposite are my favourite ways.

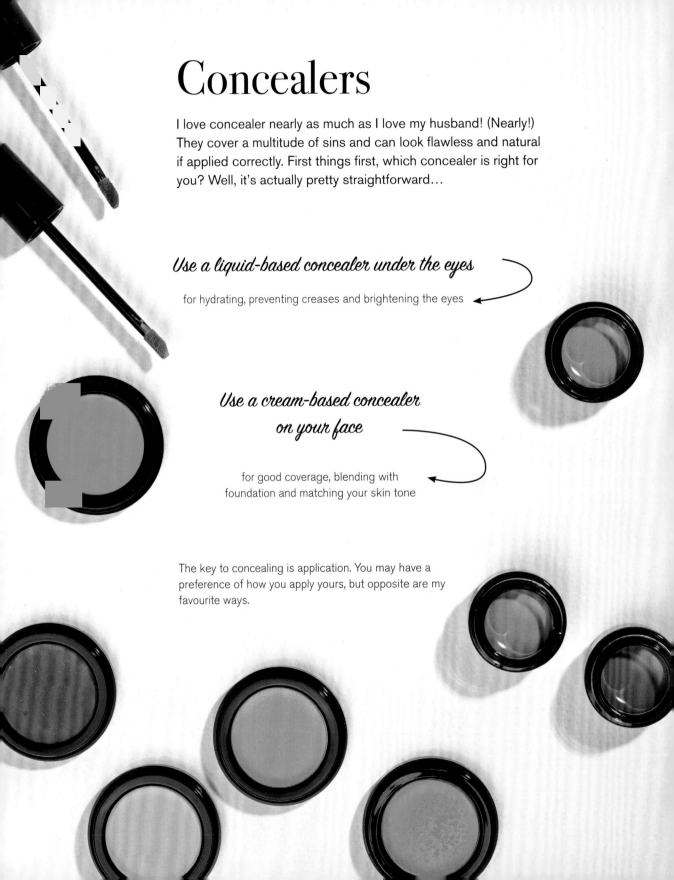

Blemishes

Whether you have one spot or ten, covering them is key. Pin-pointing is best (this is a Lisa Eldridge special), where you take a thin brush (like an eyeliner brush) and a matte cream concealer (anti-bacterial ones, such as Boi-ing by Benefit are best) and pop a touch of concealer on the spot. Next, take a clean fluffy eyeshadow brush and softly blend over the spot to give an airbrushed finish. Repeat if necessary.

Scars and pigmentation

Start with the right colour corrector for your skin tone (see right). Press this onto the problem area using your fingertips. Cover with foundation, then using a fluffy eyeshadow brush, buff concealer onto the scars or pigmentation. Stick with a matte concealer here, especially when covering scars, as a dewy concealer will only make them stand out more.

Redness

If the redness is significant, start with a yellow-based colour corrector underneath and over the top of foundation. Then take a cream concealer to match your skin tone, and press it over the top with a damp sponge. If you need to blend out the edges, use a fluffy eyeshadow brush. Blend in circular motions. Repeat if necessary.

Colour correctors

I'm a big fan of colour correctors. It's amazing how they can balance and even out the complexion. The two biggest mistakes made are, first, picking the wrong shade and second, applying so much product that you suddenly look slightly odd. (Or, if using a lavender corrector, a bit like Violet Beauregarde in Charlie and the Chocolate Factory.) So, to avoid all errors, below is a basic chart detailing which colours work for which dilemmas.

— **Redness or rosiness:** yellow corrector

— **Sallowness or yellowness:** lavender corrector

— **Dark circles, scars and pigmentation (fair to light complexion):** salmon corrector

— **Dark circles, scars and pigmentation (light to medium complexion):** peach corrector

— **Dark circles, scars and pigmentation (medium to dark complexion):** orange corrector

— **Dark circles, scars and pigmentation (dark to deep complexion):** red concealer

Rosacea and pigmentation

Once you've picked the right shade of colour corrector for your dilemma, the next step is to apply it. You can use a brush or a sponge, but I find that I get the best results when I use my fingers. The warmth of the fingers helps to blend the product onto the surface of the skin.

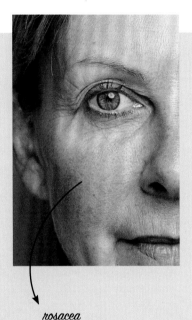

rosacea

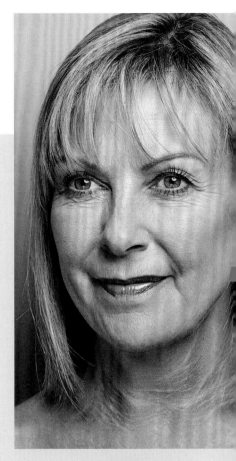

step 1 Moisturize and apply primer

step 2 Press your chosen colour corrector over the problem area with your fingertips.

step 3 Apply foundation by buffing it over the top of the colour corrector but be careful not to buff too hard.

step 4 Apply more colour corrector if needed, using fingertips again.

step 5 Blend concealer over the top of the colour corrector (see page 30), then finish the rest of your make-up.

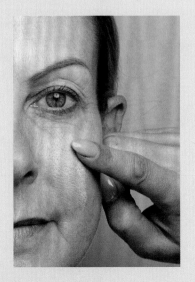

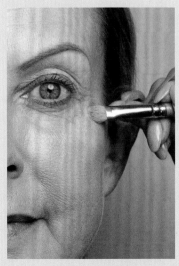

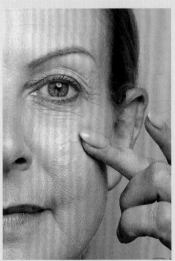

Concealer for the eyes

Brightening under your eyes with concealer makes such a huge difference to your look. If you don't have dark circles and just want to brighten under the eyes, then draw a triangle from the inner corner of the eye, down to the top of the cheek bone, up to the outer corner of the eye and blend upwards. Do this over the top of your foundation.

step 1 After your colour corrector (if needed), apply concealer by drawing a low 'V' underneath the eye. By going this low you will ensure you cover any darkness.

step 2 Apply the concealer onto the eyelid and blend down to the lash line and up to the brow with a damp sponge (I use Beautyblender®) or fluffy

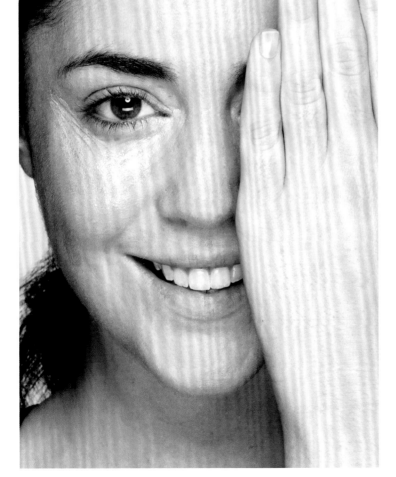

eyeshadow brush. The eye area is 40 per cent thinner than the rest of your face, so putting concealer on the lid as well as under the eye will brighten the skin for a natural finish and act as a great base for eyeshadow.

step 3 For under the eye, blend upwards with a damp sponge (it must be damp otherwise the product will not blend flawlessly).

step 4 (optional) This is a tip that I learnt from the amazing make-up artist Wayne Goss. For those seriously dark areas under the eye. Take a cotton bud/swab, dip it in concealer, spray it with a touch of water so that it's damp, then stroke it over the darkest areas under the eye. Repeat until the concealer is blended in fully.

step 5 (optional) Take a loose, lightweight translucent powder and dust it over the concealer to set it.

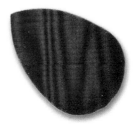

Covering dark circles

This is a beauty dilemma that many women suffer with. It can be caused by loads of things including stress, lack of sleep, dehydration or it can be hereditary. To show you the difference well-applied colour corrector and conceaer can make, I've roped in one of my oldest friends, Clare. We've been friends since we were 11 years old and Clare has always had difficulty with dark circles. It's a family trait.

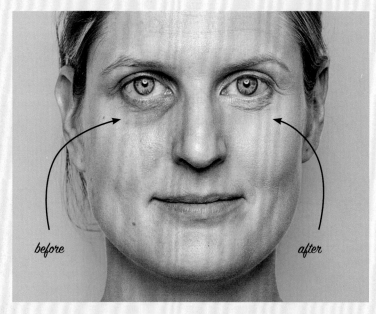

before   *after*

When I called Clare and said, 'so do you fancy showing the world your under eyes if I promise to show you how to cover them properly (oh and if I supply Prosecco)?' I wasn't quite sure what she would say. 'If it helps other women I'm in,' was her response. And Clare, I'm absolutely sure it will. So here's how to cover those pesky dark circles properly!

step 1 Begin by patting an eye cream around the orbital bone (the socket around the eye). Blend upwards towards the eye to hydrate the whole area.

step 2 Use a fluffy eyeshadow brush to buff in colour corrector.

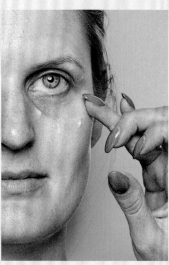
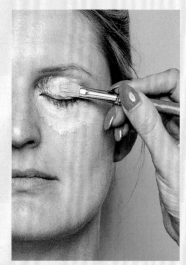
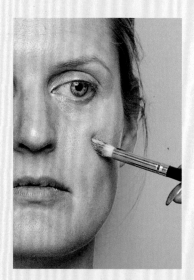

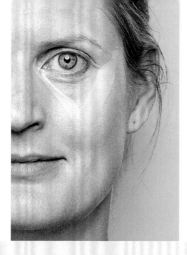
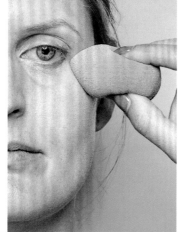
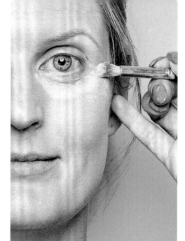

(As Clare is fair-skinned, I have used a salmon-toned corrector.) Buff this down to the top of the cheekbones (yes, that low!) and up to the brow bone, covering the entire eyelid. Add a little extra on the inner corner of the eye as it tends to be extra dark there.

step 3 Now for foundation. Buff this all over your face as usual. Be gentle when applying it over the top of the colour corrector. For a super-soft touch, use a damp sponge.

step 4 Conceal the eye area with a liquid concealer slightly brighter than your skin tone. Something yellow-based, such as Benefit's Stay Don't Stray which is my fave. Once the concealer is even, use the tip from Wayne Goss (step 4, page 33) to brighten the area around the eye.

step 5 Set the concealer with a lightweight translucent powder. I like to apply this with a damp beautyblender®. Leave for a couple of minutes to bake (this is when the powder heats up the concealer to set it), then sweep it away with a fluffy eyeshadow brush. Dark circles, gone!

How gorgeous does Clare look?

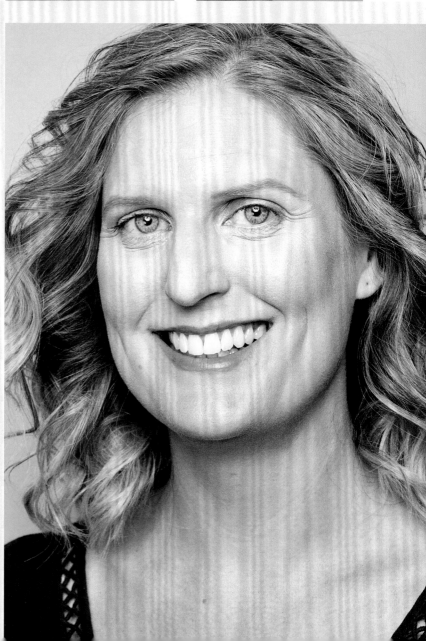

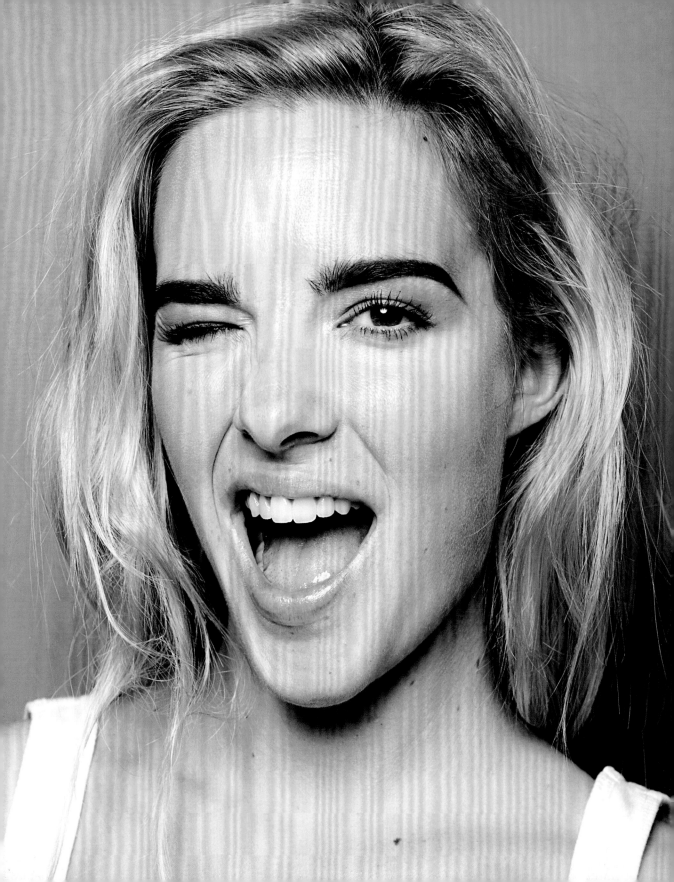

Beautiful brows

'Brushes brows, doesn't brush hair'

It's all about the brows! They make such a difference to your face. When well groomed they add structure, open your eyes and even make you look more awake. There are tonnes of treatments and styling options available that you can do at home or have done at a salon. From waxing and threading to tinting and filling, we've never paid as much attention to our brows as we do right now.

In this section, I take a look at the brow basics, which products to invest in, which treatments to have and what to do if you have troublesome eyebrows. After this, I walk you through a handful of looks that will show off your brows whatever shape or style you have.

Brow basics

I love eyebrows. A well-groomed, defined brow can be as powerful as an eye lift (without the injections)! They can change your look and your face more than any make-up product. Neat brows are my biggest 'hide-the-hangover', tired-eyes tip because they make you look more awake, instantly.

Like us, eyebrows come in all shapes and sizes. From bushy to sparse, holey and scarred, to more tadpole than tamed. Don't despair, there's always a solution to help you groom your ultimate brow.

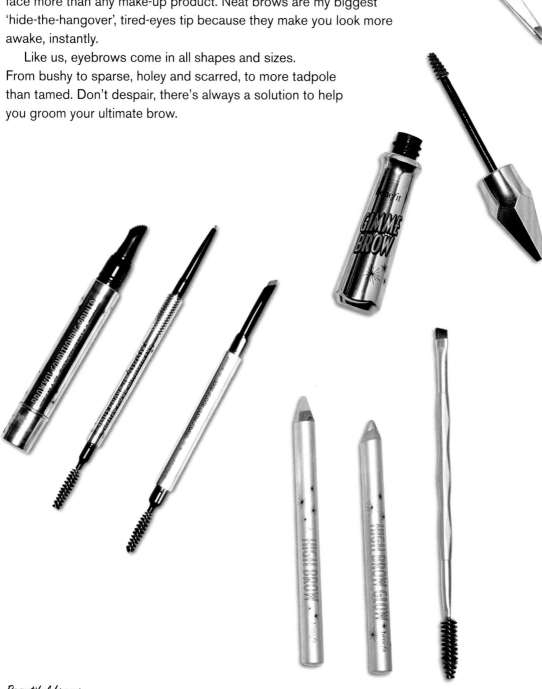

Brow treatments

If you've never had your brows professionally shaped then put this book down, get on the blower ('phone' for those across the pond) and book an appointment immediately! No matter how good you think you are at tweezing your own brows, the professionals will always do it that little bit better!

Waxing

My favourite brow treatment, without a doubt, is waxing. I'm a wimp. Any type of hair removal makes me as dramatic as a soap-opera character that's just found out that their next-door neighbour is actually their mother! And that's exactly why I like waxing – it's quick. Full stop. Added to that, it's precise and gives a clean finish.

Threading

Threading can be amazing if you find the right person to do it and aren't as much as a wimp as me! It's an ancient art form and many people swear by it. For me, it's just too speedy. I always panic that a wrong hair might be removed by mistake. And one wrong hair taken from your brow is comparable to shaving off half of the hair on your head, right?! (Well, it is in my mind.)

Tinting

I wouldn't have my brows waxed without having them tinted, even though my natural brow colour is dark brown. (Although I've had them tinted for so many years that they could be blonde for all I know!) A brow tint makes your brows look fuller and healthier no matter your brow shape or colour. It takes about three minutes and lasts about six weeks – it's a no-brainer.

Tattooing

If I'd been writing this book ten years ago, I would have told you to avoid tattooing at all cost! However, technology has changed and now there are some incredible brow artists out there. This can be the perfect treatment for someone whose brows are non-existent whether that's the result of over-plucking or alopecia, or a side-effect of medical treatment. If this is the right choice for you, then do your research. You want an artist who creates hair-like stokes with the tattoo-gun, not one who block-draws. My aunt recently had this done and it's made an incredible difference to her face and to her confidence. So it can definitely be worth the money and time. But remember, it's permanent so make sure that it's right for you before you go for it.

Micro-blading

This is a relatively new technique. Micro-blading is a semi-permanent treatment that tends to last between 18 and 36 months. It's a manual technique where a tiny, handheld micro-blade deposits the pigment into the superficial dermis of the skin. The results can be amazing if you have very sparse brows, but again, this is a big decision with a pretty hefty price tag so I'd try waxing and tinting before you make up your mind.

Brow mapping

I first learnt about brows working at Benefit. They are the brow authority, without a doubt, and have been shaping and styling brows since 1976. Their mapping technique works for everyone and makes your brows the best they can be. So, let's start there. Grab a mirror, a make-up brush and your favourite brow product. And let's map!

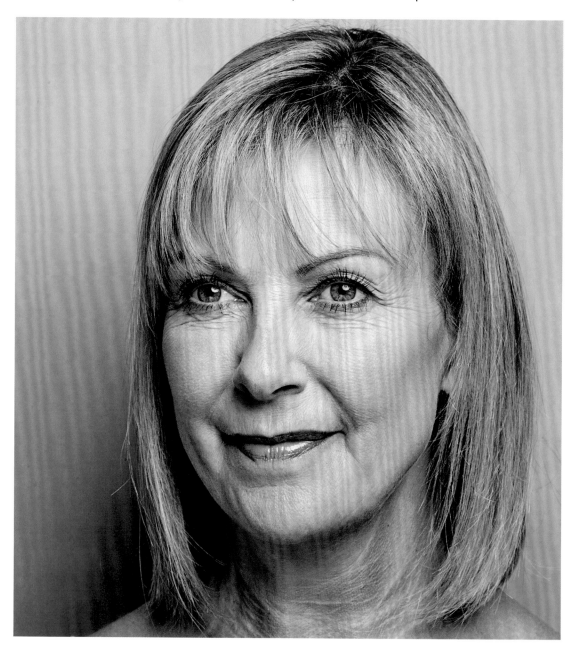

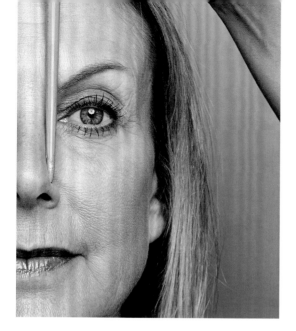

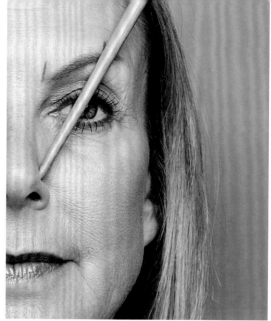

step 1 Look straight ahead into a mirror. Hold the brush from the dimple of your nose, straight up to your brow. Mark a line using a brow product. Starting your brow here will make your nose look slimmer.

step 2 Hold the brush at the dimple of the nose and straight through your pupil to find the arch. Make sure you're looking straight ahead and mark this point. Positioning your arch in the right place will give an instant eye lift.

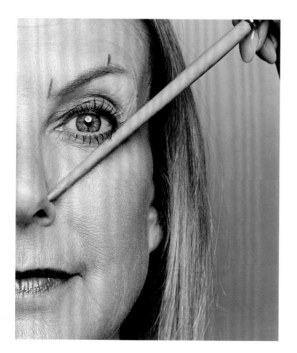

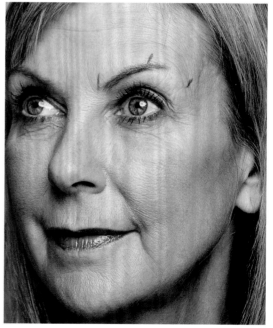

step 3 Hold the brush at the dimple of your nose through the outer corner of the eye, up to the brow. Mark this point. Ending your brow in the right place will lift your cheekbones.

step 4 Now that you have perfectly mapped brows you can fill them in. Over the next few pages I show you how to get different brow styles and how to solve different brow dilemmas, but these are the basics.

Natural brows

Enhancing your brows is quick and easy and will lift your whole look. For this natural look, I use a brow fibre gel. These products mimic the appearance of real hair and work well alone or over the top of any other brow product. This is also pretty foolproof, I promise!

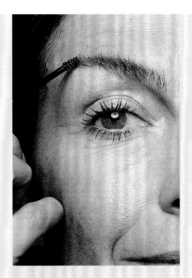

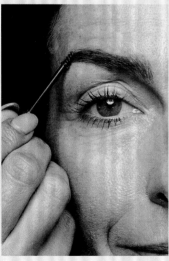

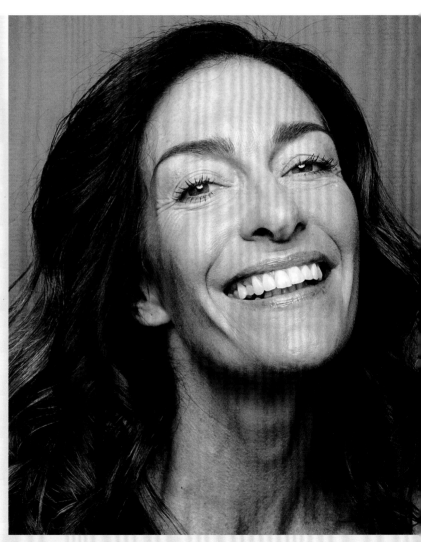

step 1 Brush away from the brow hair first, using the brow fibre gel.

step 2 Brush back in the same direction as the hair. This will coat each hair from root to tip, making the most of the product.

step 3 (optional) Create an instant eye lift by drawing a line beneath them with a brow highlighter pencil. And blend!

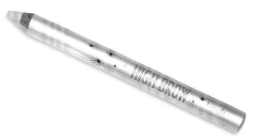

all you need...

brow fibre gel

brow highlighter
pencil (optional)

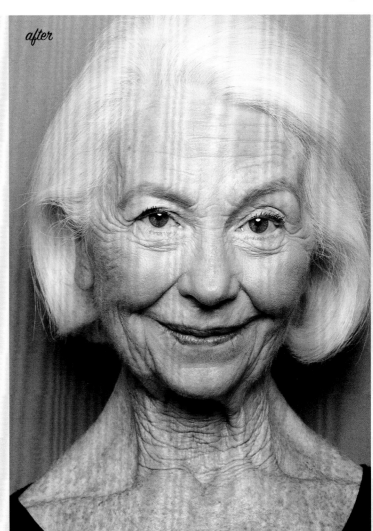

before

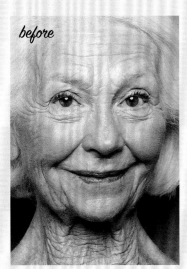

*If you are worried about colouring
in your eyebrows because you
have fair hair, don't be.
Look how great it looks!*

Defined brows

Sometimes eyebrows have very little shape or have been over-plucked meaning that they are not the shape that we want them to be. If you're confident with make-up, you can absolutely draw a full, arched brow in using brow products. However, this takes time and, if done wrong, can make you look like you've 'stuck' your brow on. So this look will define your brows and make them look thicker, without going OTT.

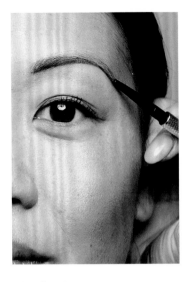

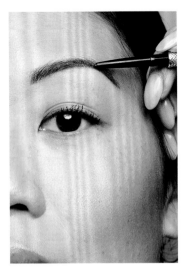

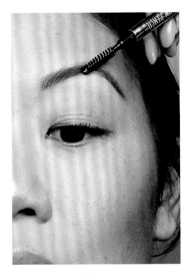

step 1 Map your brows so you know where they should start, arch and end (see pages 40–41). Using a sharp brow pencil, draw a line slightly under your natural arch. This will add definition and make your brows look slightly thicker and more defined.

step 2 Fill in your brow with the brow pencil, using hair like strokes to give a natural look.

step 3 Brush through the brow with a brow brush. (All good brow pencils have these on the end of them.) Brushing through the brow will soften and even out any areas where you may have applied too much product.

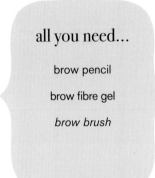

all you need...

brow pencil

brow fibre gel

brow brush

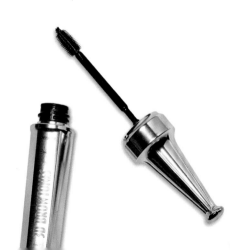

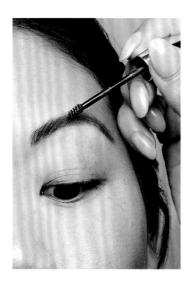

step 4 Brow fibre gels are the best invention EVER! They make your brows look fuller and thicker instantly due to the clever micro-fibres in the formula. Brush against the hair first to coat the underneath of the hairs. (Think of this as like back-combing the hair on the end.)

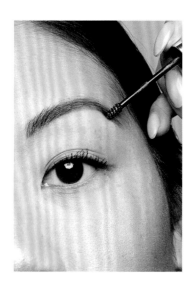

step 5 Brush the fibre gel through the brow in the direction of the hair growth. This will coat the top of the hair and keep your brows in place.

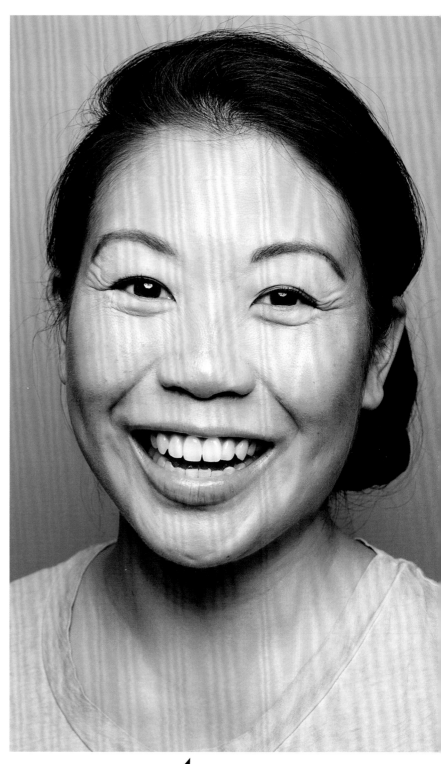

Defined brows, complete!

Bold brows

When I talk about 'bold' brows, I don't mean crazy, stuck-on, comedy brows. I mean full, groomed, power brows. Anyone can have bold brows, whether you have the hair there or not. Although bold brows don't suit everyone. For this look I've used a cream gel brow product because I find this easy to control, buildable and long-wearing.

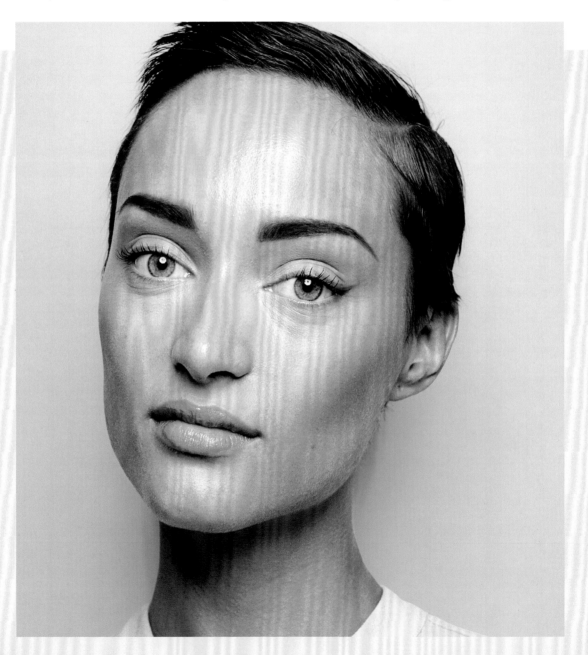

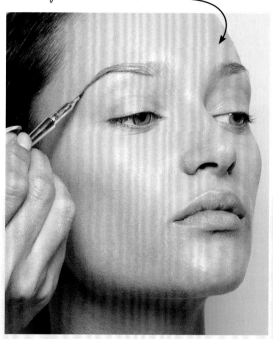

note how fair her natural brows are

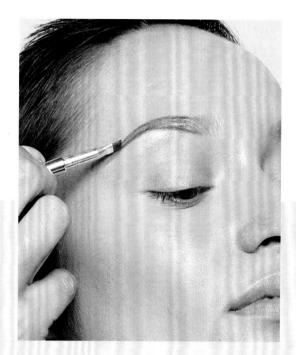

step 1 Map your brows so you know where they should start, arch and end (see pages 40–41). Draw a fluid line using a cream gel brow product and a thin brow brush slightly underneath the brow arch. This will give the brow a bit of extra width whilst still holding the shape. Avoid the front section of the brow as keeping this section soft is the key to a good bold brow.

step 2 (optional) Using the same product and brush, draw a fluid line on top of the brow. Going slightly above the hair line will give you a fuller looking brow. If you want a softer finish, avoid the top line.

all you need...

cream gel brow product

brow spoolie

brow brush

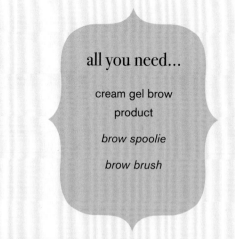

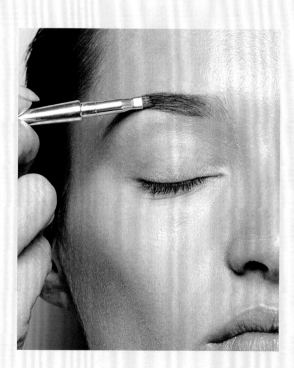

step 3 Fill in the brow using the flat side of the brush, avoiding the front section.

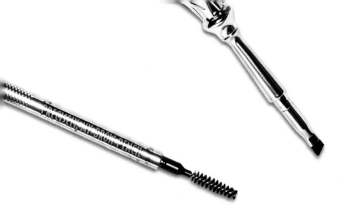

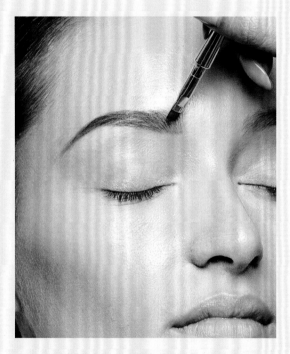

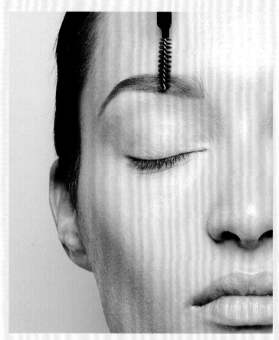

step 4 Without dipping the brush back into the product, run the brush upwards through the front of the brow. This will add a small amount of product into this section.

step 5 Brush through the brow with a brow spoolie to blend the colour through.

Top tip

The darker the brow shade you use, the bolder the brows will look.

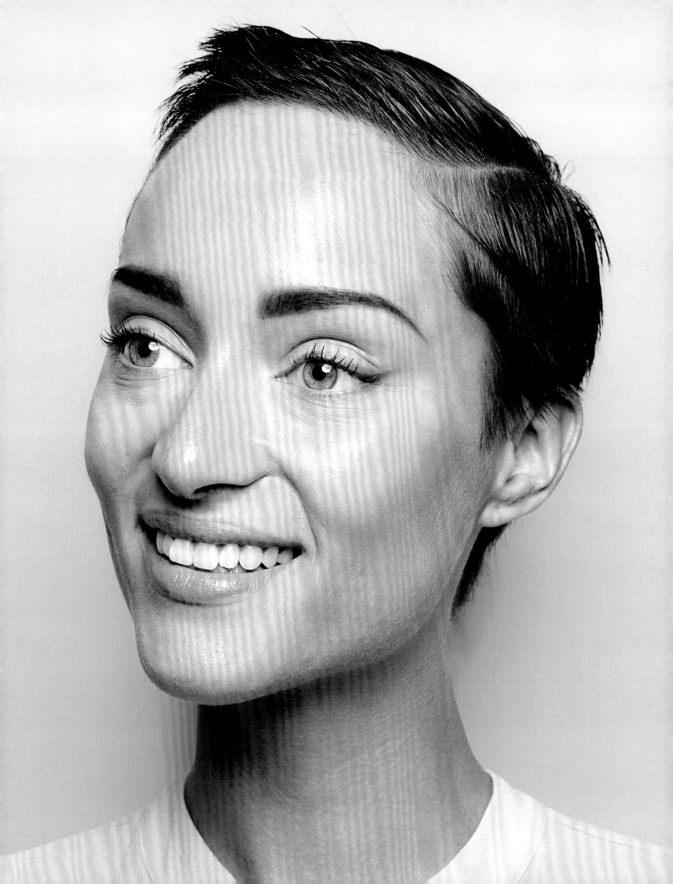

Hair today-gone tomorrow!

It's a well known fact that as we get older, our eyebrows become more sparse. Unlike men, whose eyebrows continue to grow like wildfire! Losing the tail of the brow can change the look of your face, so drawing it back in is a must. Certain illnesses and treatments can also cause hair loss, so this is a great way to get your brows back.

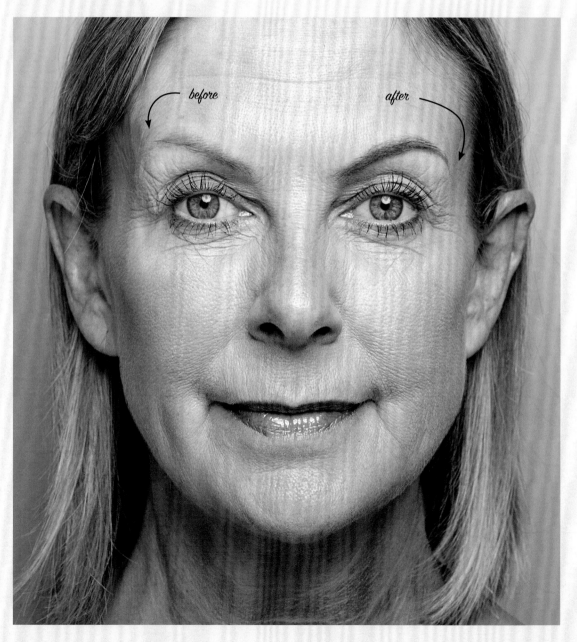

before

after

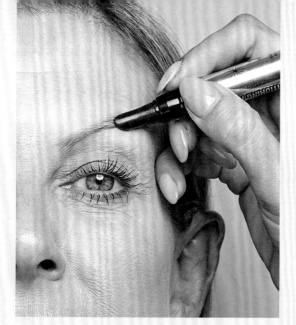

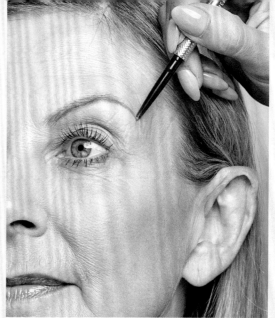

step 1 Use a brow conditioning primer, morning and night. This will help to make your brow hair look healthier and fuller. Build this into your skincare routine.

step 2 Map your brows so you know where they should start, arch and end (see pages 40–41). Use a pencil that adheres to skin as well as hair. My favourite is Benefit's Precisely My Brow pencil as it has an ultra-fine tip and 12-hour waterproof wear. Fill in your brow, extending it to the correct point.

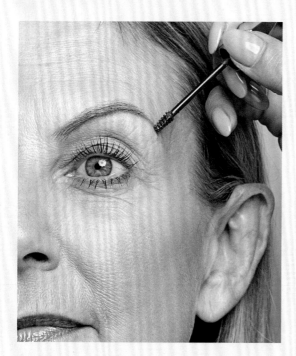

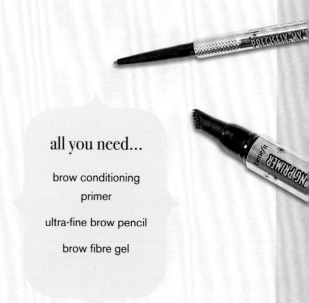

all you need...

brow conditioning primer

ultra-fine brow pencil

brow fibre gel

step 3 To add volume, use a fibre gel on the brows to go away from the hair, then back with the hair. This will make the drawn-in section of the brow look more like hair as it has micro fibres in it, which mimic the appearance of real hair. Your brows should now be well and truly back where they should be!

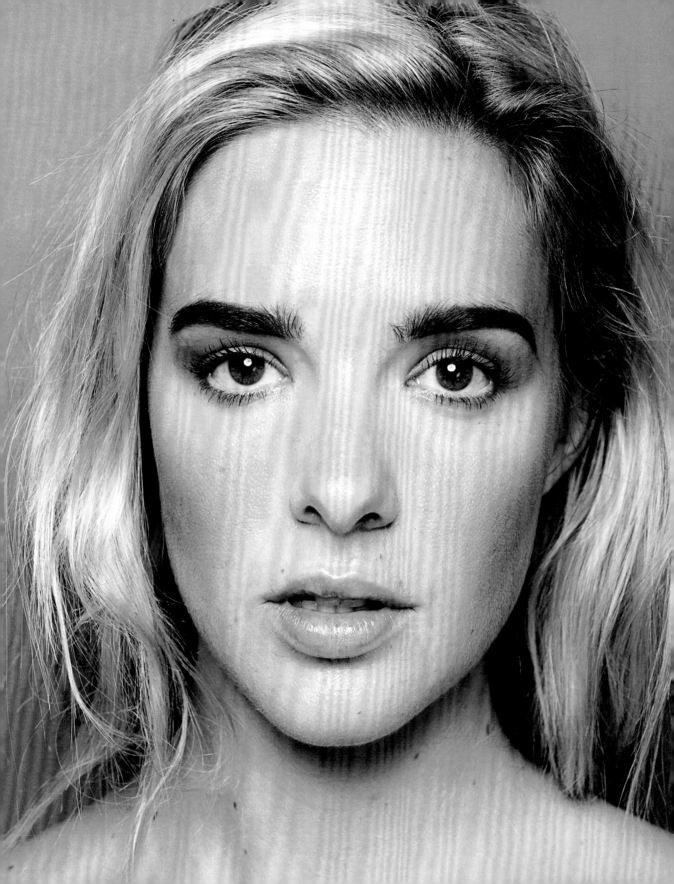

Feathered brows

A feathered brow is a cool alternative to a bold brow. It's slightly softer and can add edge to your overall look.

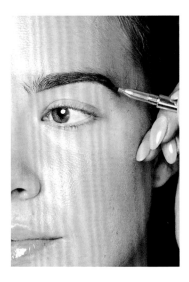

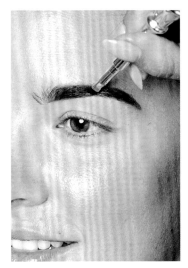

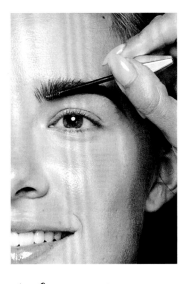

step 1 Map your brows so you know where they should start, arch and end (see pages 40–41). Draw a fluid line under the brow, using an brow gel, avoiding the front of the eyebrow. We'll be using a different product there as we don't want to add too much weight to the front as this can make the brow look stuck on.

step 2 Fill in the brow, using the same product and the flat side of the brush, again avoiding the front section.

step 3 Use a brow fibre gel brush through the brow to mimic the appearance of real hair. Brush through the entire eyebrow, including the front. If your hair allows it, brush the front up slightly for a feathered look. If you don't have hair that looks right brushed up at the front, then use an ultra-fine brow pencil to draw hairs upwards at the front of the brow.

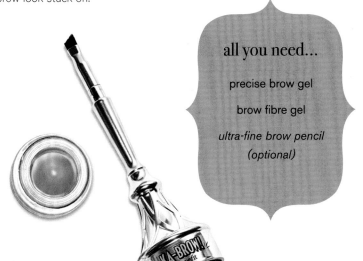

all you need...

precise brow gel

brow fibre gel

*ultra-fine brow pencil
(optional)*

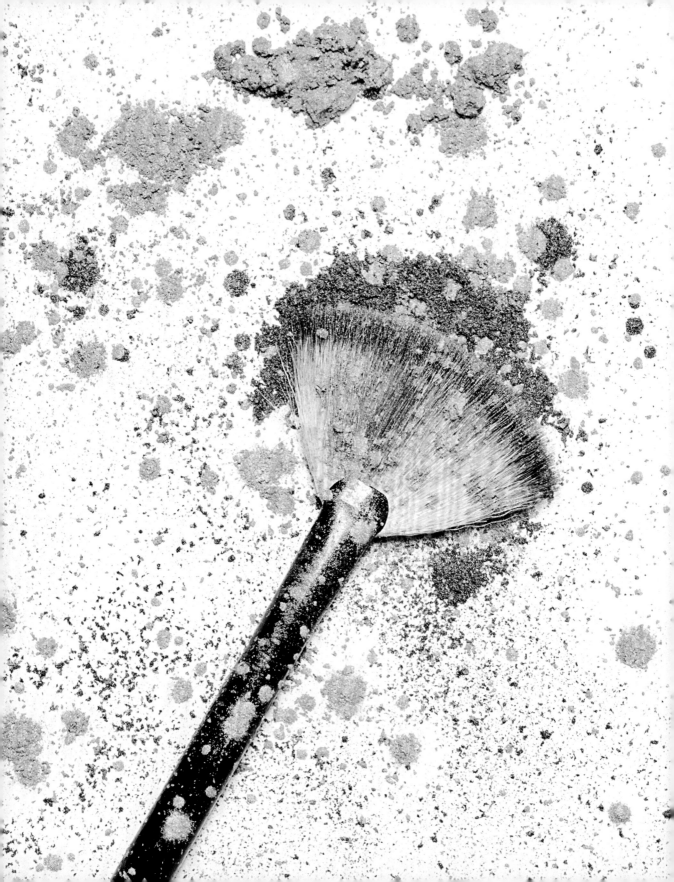

Go with the glow

This chapter is all about colour. And I love colour! You know that feeling at the height of summer when you feel like you look really healthy, sunkissed and just plain gorgeous? Well, it doesn't have to be just once a year.

Whether it's a lick of blusher over the cheeks to give you a light flush or full-on contouring with bronzers galore, you'll know exactly where to put the pop to look your best. This is where make-up artists can really transform a look by manipulating the base to add shape and definition to the face. I discuss strobing and bronzing and all that's in between with a handful of looks that show off colour best.

For all you need to know about blusher, bronzer, contouring and highlighting...

Blusher basics

The combination of bronzer, blusher and highlighter can make you look healthier, it can define the structure of your face and add a youthful glow to your look. I know you're all flicking ahead thinking, 'How? Tell me, quick!' However, these are the three things that are also very easy to get wrong, but not anymore with these basics.

Types of blusher

A pop of blusher adds colour and dimension to your look. There are so many colours and types of blushers to choose from so I'm going to break it down for you.

Powder

These work on the majority of skin types, apart from super-dry ones. They are fab because you can build and blend them to perfection. Powder blusher also works with all foundation types.

Cream

I love how cream blusher blends into your complexion seamlessly and how it adds a sheen to your skin. They work on all skin types apart from oily skin. They also work best with liquid and cream-based foundations.

Stains and gels

These are fab for long wear, giving a natural glow. They are more difficult to blend than the alternatives. But can look fab all day long once applied. They work best with a liquid foundation.

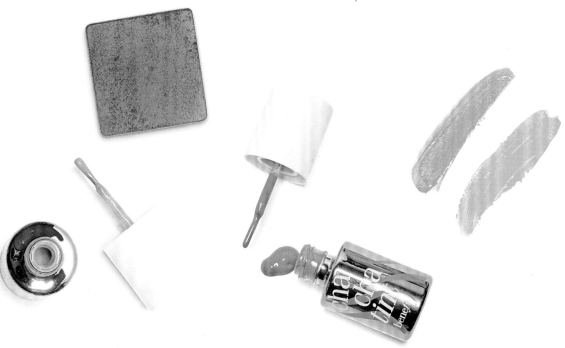

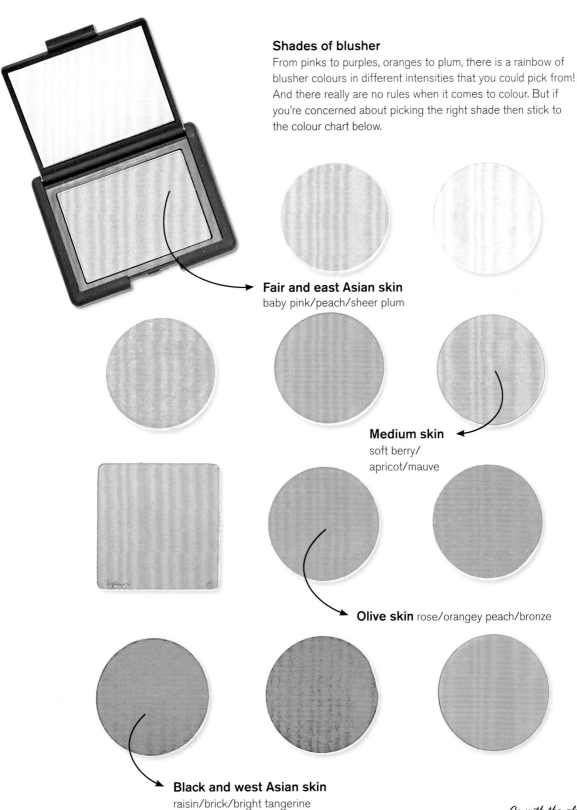

Shades of blusher

From pinks to purples, oranges to plum, there is a rainbow of blusher colours in different intensities that you could pick from! And there really are no rules when it comes to colour. But if you're concerned about picking the right shade then stick to the colour chart below.

Fair and east Asian skin
baby pink/peach/sheer plum

Medium skin
soft berry/
apricot/mauve

Olive skin rose/orangey peach/bronze

Black and west Asian skin
raisin/brick/bright tangerine

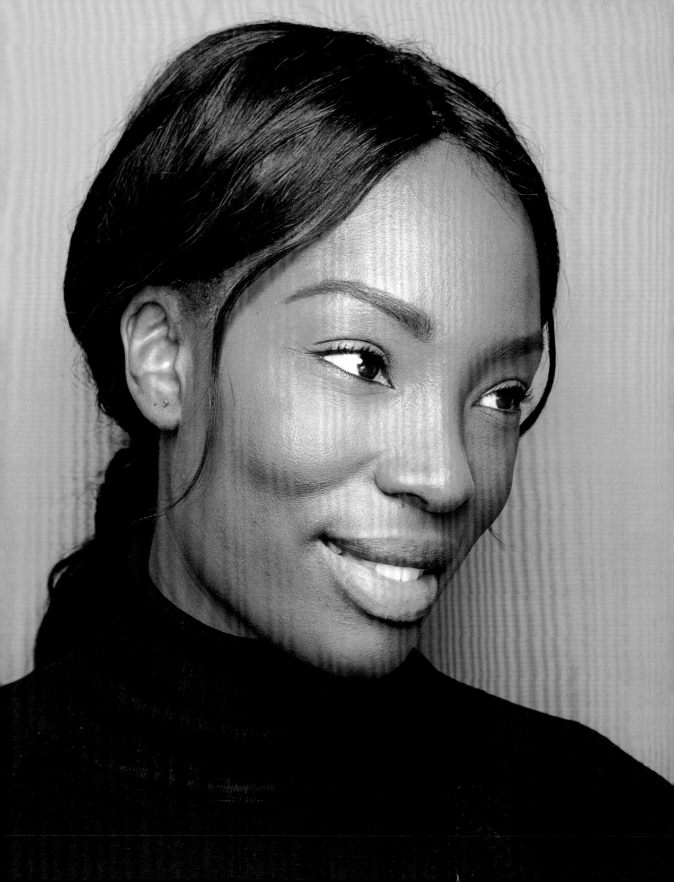

Where to put the pop

If you're unsure of where to position your blusher to enhance your face shape then here's a little guide. For creams, stains and gels, I recommend patting them in place with your fingers. For powders, a small–medium head blusher brush is best.

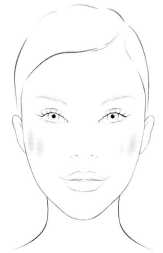

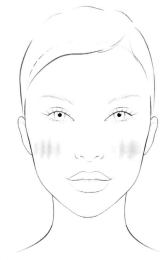

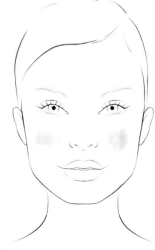

Oval face
Any application works, but to keep the face balanced, start in the middle of the apples of the cheeks and sweep upwards towards the temples.

Heart face
To soften the look of the jawline, bring focus to your cheeks by softly blending blusher just on the apples of your cheeks.

Square face
Similar to a heart shape, soften the look of your jaw by focusing the blush onto the apples of the cheeks. Blend softly with your blusher brush.

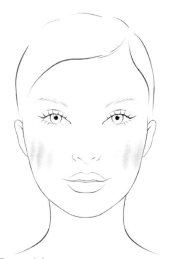

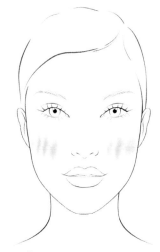

Always start with a smile as that will reveal the apples of your cheeks!

Round face
Start on the apples of your cheeks and sweep upwards towards the top of the ears to create definition.

Long face
Create width by sweeping blusher outwards from the apples, across the cheeks horizontally.

Brushes

Hands up if you have 50 make up brushes and no idea what to do with half of them… I know this is the scenario for most of my friends. The other extreme is that you only have one brush that you use for literally EVERYTHING! Foundation, cheeks, lips, eyes – everything! Well, the reality is that you only need a handful of brushes. Here are the key types of brush with a brief descripton of what they do. The ones with the gold stars next to them are the ones that in my opinion, everyone needs in their make-up kit.

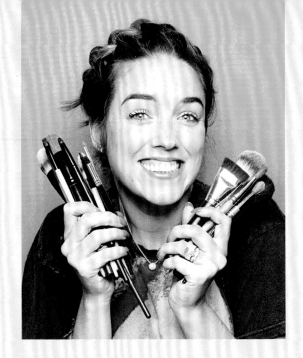

Fluffy eyeshadow brush
I have about 50 fluffy eyeshadow brushes. I suggest you have two or three of these. Particularly if you wear a lot of eyeshadow. They are great for applying and blending all different types of eyeshadows. I always use at least two of these brushes when creating a smokey eye: one to apply the product and a clean one to buff in the shadow, particularly when using colour as I find these need more buffing to get an even finish.

I also LOVE these brushes for applying concealer and, if I have time, foundation – buffing in small round circular motions will give you the most perfect base (see page 28). Yes it takes time, but it's worth it!

Oh and they are great for applying and blending highlighters too!

Pencil brush
Great for smudging liners and for smudging and blending shadow under the eyes. These are fab for precision-blending on the eye (like in a Cut Crease look, see pages 110–113). If you want a stained lip look, use this brush to softly rub in your lipstick.

Fluffy contour brush
These brushes are great for blending, particularly if you have round or almond-shaped eyes. They are not as precise as a fluffy eyeshadow brush due to the size of the head, but they are great for a smokey eye.

Lip brush
There are loads of different shapes and size of lip brushes and picking the right one really depends on your lip shape. I like a round, thin shape tip as I find it works well for all lip shapes and is tapered enough to define the lip line.

Hard-angle brush
These are generally used for eyebrows. They are perfect for this. But they can also be used on lips and for lining eyes, perfect for multiple use!

Foundation brush
No prizes for guessing what this brush is for! You need this brush if you prefer to use a brush to apply your base. I personally prefer to use my fingers, a beauty blender or a fluffy eyeshadow brush as I sometimes find that foundation brushes can cause streaks. Kabuki brushes are also great for applying powder foundation.

Contour bronzer brush
If you love wearing bronzer then this type of tapered brush is awesome. It really gets into the hollows of the cheeks. You can also use it for applying blusher.

Blusher brush
A lot of blushers come with mini brushes for on the go, but for a beautiful, blended blusher look, a full-size brush is key. These also work for blending foundation.

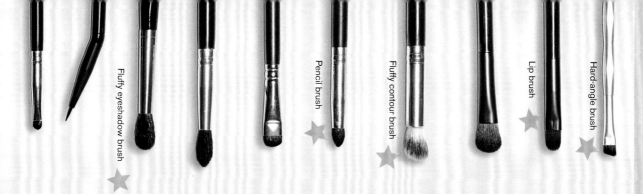

Fluffy eyeshadow brush

Pencil brush

Fluffy contour brush

Lip brush

Hard-angle brush

Other tools I love

Beauty blender
These are a type of sponge. They are amazing for applying your base, concealer, cream blushers and powder. I like to dampen them before use as this tends to give an airbrushed finish, whatever you are doing.

Fantail brush (see picture on page 54)
I use these to apply powder, highlighter and a light touch of blusher or bronzer.

Tweezers
I'm obsessed! I love Tweezerman tweezers as they are so sharp and precise, and come with a warranty that means you can send them off for sharpening for free.

Pencil sharpener
I always carry three sharpeners in my kit as it's one of those things you can never find when you need it!

Cotton bud/swab
The pointy ones are the best for precisely removing or blending make-up.

Cleaning brushes

I clean my brushes every single day, as well as cleaning them throughout my working day. But that's because I need to as I'm working on different faces and creating different looks all the time.

If you're only using your brushes on yourself then I would try to clean them as often as possible – once a week is ideal. Or before each new make-up look (especially when it comes to applying eyeshadow).

My Sigma Spa® brush-cleaning glove is my everything! Mainly because it helps me to clean my brushes so quickly. (It costs around £30/$40 to buy.) A sheet of Lego® can also do the trick (you know the big, flat bit you build stuff on top of). Just rinse your brush and rub the head over the Lego® with a bit of brush cleaner or shampoo, then rinse! (Who knew Lego® could be so useful!)

Talking of cleaning. Using your own hair shampoo works well when picking a cleaning product. You know you're not allergic to it and it will clean the brush well, just like it does the hair on your head. I always double clean my brush, then leave them to dry naturally on a towel overnight. Don't put them near direct heat as the glue that holds the bristles could melt. There are also loads of brush cleaners out there. The quick-drying ones are the best as you can use the brushes again after a few minutes. Just remember, if you don't clean your brushes regularly, you're prone to infection. Nobody wants that, so make sure you clean those babies!

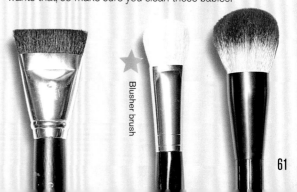

Foundation brush

Contour bronzer brush

Blusher brush

Illuminations!

Highlighter has always been a key product in my kit. There are so many to choose from and my problem is that I love them all! I love to layer them to channel a disco ball!

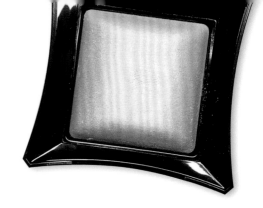

Types of highlighter

Liquid
This is my fave type of highlighter, mainly because it blends so beautifully. It looks great mixed with foundation or applied to the highpoints of the face.

Cream
Cream highlighters are my fashion-week faves. They are quick and tend to have a stronger glow than liquid. Cream highlighters also look amazing down the centre of the legs, on the collar bone and on the shoulders.

Powder
These give that finishing touch. I love layering a powder over a cream or liquid to intensify the glow.

Picking the right shade

There are an array of highlighter shades, you can even buy rainbow highlighters! However, if you want to look less unicorn and more angel, stick to the shades here.

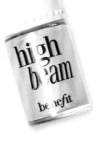

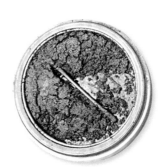

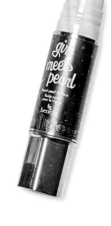

Fair skin pearls and pinks

Black skin golds and bronzes

Medium to olive skin
Champagnes and rose golds

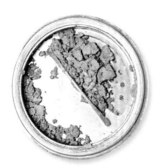

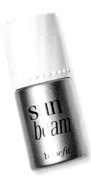

Applying highlighter

These are my two favourite ways to apply highlighter.

option 1 Mix a liquid highlighter with your liquid foundation and blend all over the face. (This is strobing territory, the ultimate highlighting. To see how to strobe check out my YouTube channel where I explain strobing and chroming and all the other 'ings'.)

option 2 Apply your chosen highlighter to the high points of your face (under your brow bones, on the cheekbones, down the nose and on the cupid's bow) and blend. This will add structure to your face as these are the areas that the light hits first.

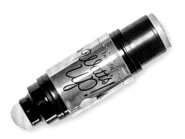

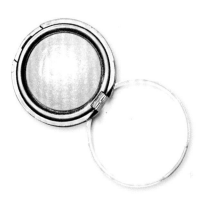

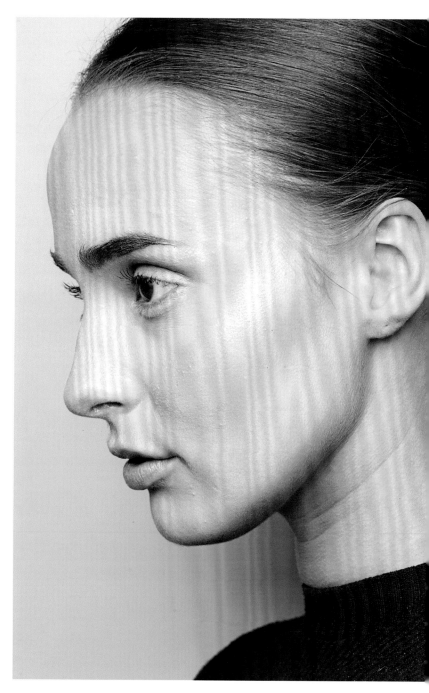

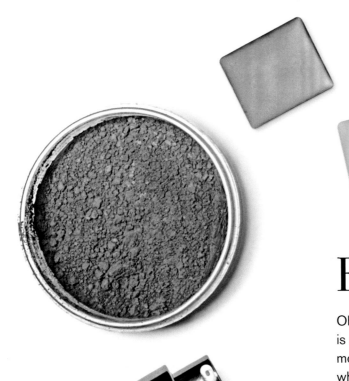

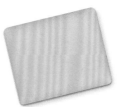

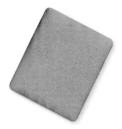

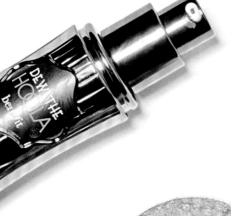

Bronzer

Oh bronzer, you lovely, lovely product. Bronzer is my 'it's going to be alright' product. I wear it most days but it is particularly useful on days where I'm not feeling my best – it just seems to perk you up like a strong cup of coffee!

Types of bronzer

Picking the right shade and texture is essential. It's easy to look muddy or orange if the wrong product is picked and I'm sure that's not the look you desire! In terms of texture, here are the options.

Powder
My fave type of bronzer. Powders are great as they blend in well and give a natural finish. The key is to apply them properly. Stick to matte types rather than ones with shimmer in. Leave the shine for the highlight.

Cream
Slightly more effort to apply, but great for contouring. Cream bronzers blend beautifully and can give you a lovely sheen.

Liquid or gel
These are great for an all-over glow. Pat them over your foundation, or mix them together with your foundation (if liquid) for a lightweight bronze.

Top tip

'Sunkissed not sunburnt!' is your mantra. The general rule when picking your bronzer shade is that it is best to go 1–2 shades darker than your natural skin tone. It's as simple as that!

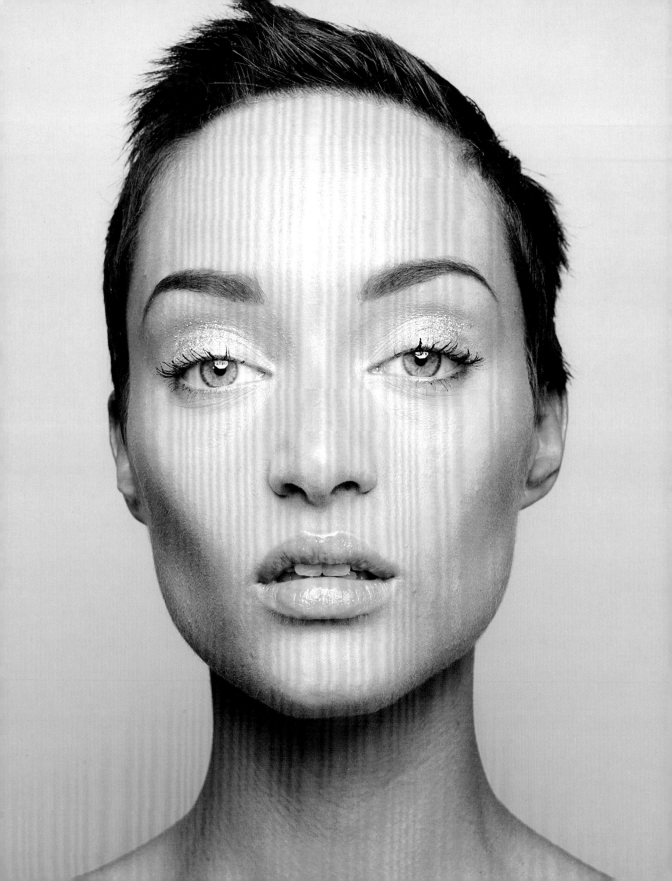

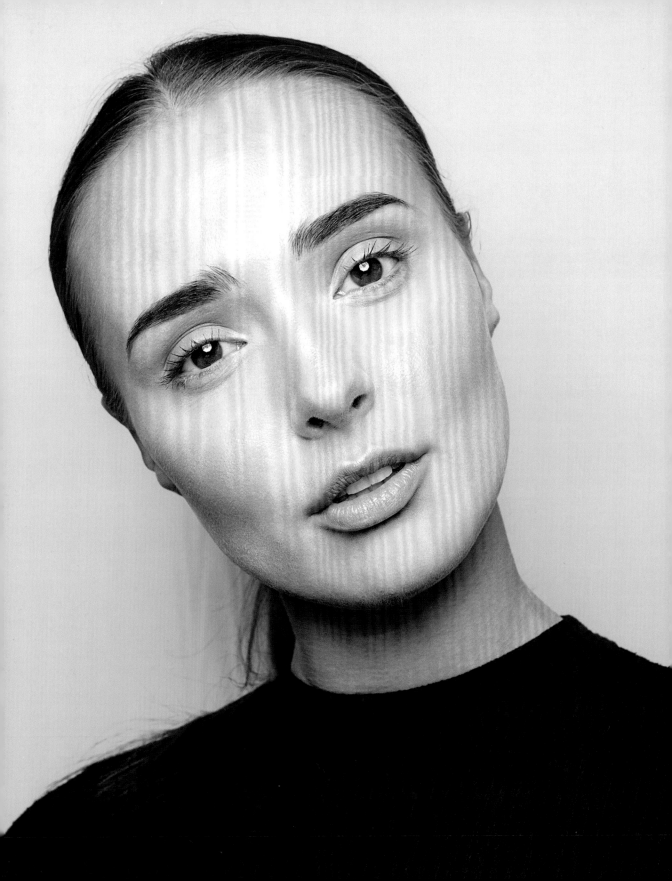

Full contour

Okay, are you ready for this? This is the ultimate contouring technique. The idea is that you highlight the areas that you want to come towards other people and bronze the areas you want to recede away. The combination of the two enhances your face structure.

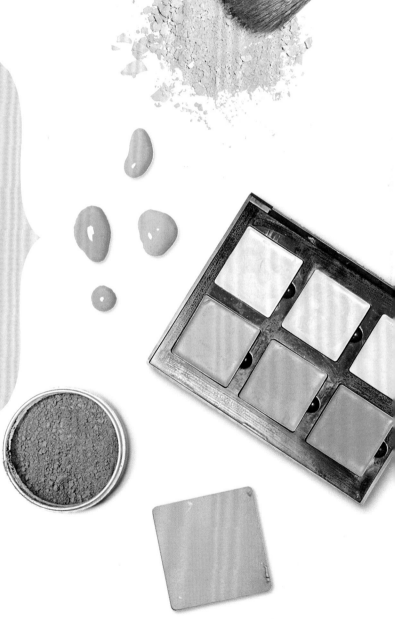

all you need...

cream bronzer
(2 shades darker than your skin tone)

cream foundation
(1 shade lighter than your skin tone)

liquid foundation
(1 shade darker than your skin tone)

loose translucent foundation powder

matte powder bronzer

powder highlighter

powder blusher

foundation brush

fluffy eyeshadow brush

fantail brush

Full contouring can look heavy in real life, but awesome in photos. Be prepared for that.

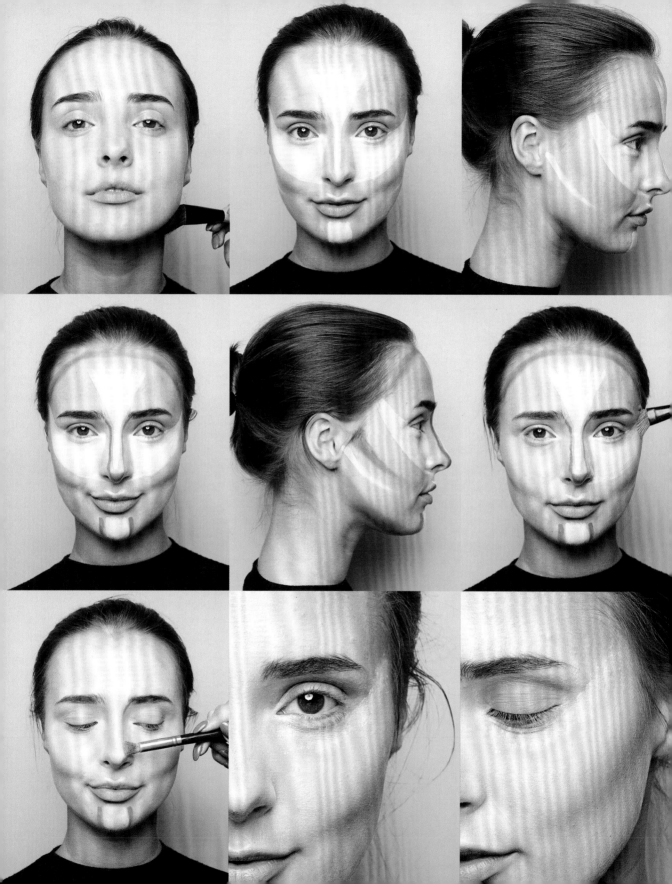

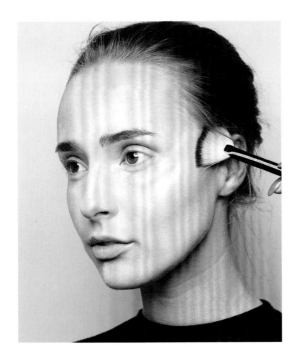
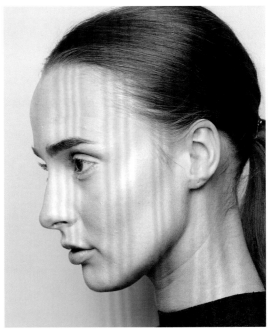

step 1 (top row, left) Moisturize the skin and sweep the matte powder bronzer down your neck and across the collarbone.

step 2 (top row, centre and right) With the light cream foundation and using a foundation brush, highlight the centre of the forehead, the bridge of the nose, the chin, under the eyes and under the cheekbones.

step 3 (middle row, left and centre) With the cream bronzer and using a fluffy eyeshadow brush, contour under the cheekbones, jaw line, hair line, temples, down the sides of the nose and in the eye sockets.

step 4 (middle row right and bottom row, left) With the liquid foundation and a fluffy blusher brush, blend the foundation over the top of everything. Blend in the direction that you applied the contour and highlight so that you don't lose the definition that you've created.

step 5 (bottom row, centre) Set under the eyes and the chin with loose powder using a fluffy eyeshadow brush. Leave it in place while you complete the next step.

step 6 (bottom row, right) With a matte powder bronzer and using a fluffy eyeshadow brush, contour under the cheekbones, jaw line, temples and eye socket.

step 7 (this page, left) Apply powder highlighter using a fantail brush under the brow bone, on top of the cheek bones and on the cupid's bow.

step 8 (this page, right) Sweep away the loose powder under the eye, add a pop of blusher and finish the rest of your make-up.

Natural contour

There are a few ways to wear bronzer. And, yes, a full contour is one of them. However, this isn't necessarily something that you'd want to do every day, or perhaps at all, because it is quite heavy. So this is my guide to a quick, everyday, natural contour that works for all ages.

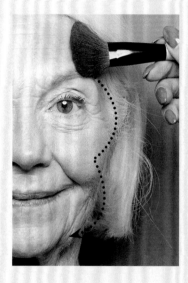

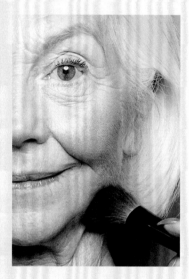

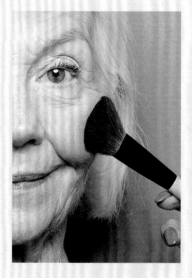

step 1 After you've completed your base. Take a matte powder bronzer and sweep it in a figure of '3' either side of the face using a blusher brush (or fantail brush for a lighter touch), starting at the forehead, working down to the cheekbones and down to the chin.

step 2 Sweep the bronzer down your neck to match it to your face.

step 3 Add a pop of blusher to the cheeks and highlight the high points of your face with highlighter and a blusher brush.

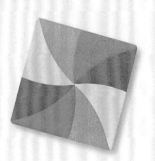

all you need...

matte powder bronzer

highlighter

blusher

blusher or fantail brush

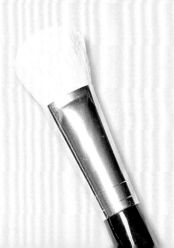

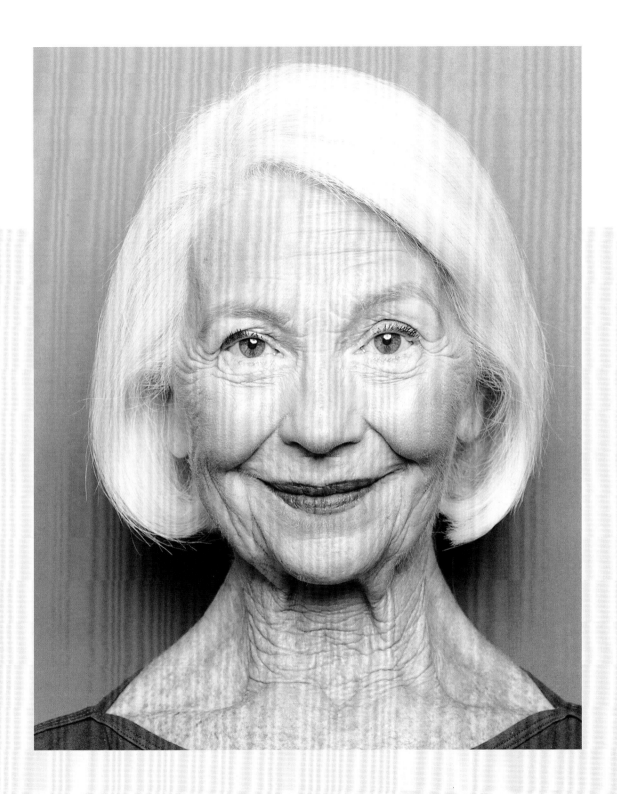

From pasty to tasty!

Sunkissed skin and a golden glow are the two things that make you look and feel healthier. However, with the amount of SPF I smoother over my face, I'd be lucky to leave a sunglass mark. And that's absolutely fine by me because, as much as I love the sun it can cause premature ageing and sunspots and those are two things that I certainly want to avoid!

Luckily there are plenty of amazing bronzing products out there that can fake a tan in seconds. This look is one of my absolute favourites for summer. It's quick, easy and makes you look like a golden goddess. Pair it with wet waves for the ultimate beach babe vibe.

Perfect your base and brows before you start the steps and be sure to use a liquid foundation.

all you need...

liquid bronzer

matte powder bronzer

blusher

metallic bronze eyeshadow

metallic powder highlighter

clear lip gloss

blusher brush

fluffy eyeshadow brush

lip brush

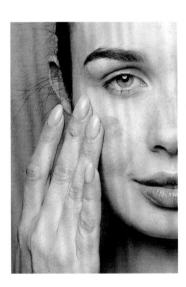

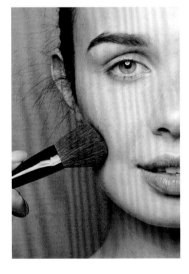

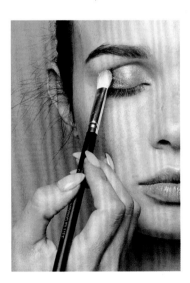

step 1 Pat a liquid bronzer all on your face and neck over your foundation. (These products are fab for giving an all-over, lightweight, warm glow.)

step 2 Sweep a matte powder bronzer either side of the face in a figure of '3', down the nose and down the neck using a blusher brush. Don't be tempted to chuck it on in any old direction. My '3' technique will define and sculpt the face, as well as looking natural. Add a pop of blusher to the apples of your cheeks with a blusher brush.

step 3 Buff a metallic bronze eyeshadow all over the eyelid, up and into the socket using a fluffy eyeshadow brush. Don't layer the shadow too much as this is more a wash of colour rather than a smokey eye. Add lots of black mascara to upper and lower lashes.

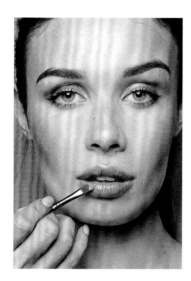

step 4 This is my favourite part. Dust a metallic powder highlighter across the highest points of your face, these being your cheek bones, brow bones, down the centre of your nose and on your cupid's bow. This adds a luminosity that really brings the look together. (It also makes your skin look incredible in pictures!)

step 5 Use a lip brush or your ring finger to press the metallic powder highlighter into the centre of your lips. Finish by applying a clear lip gloss over the top.

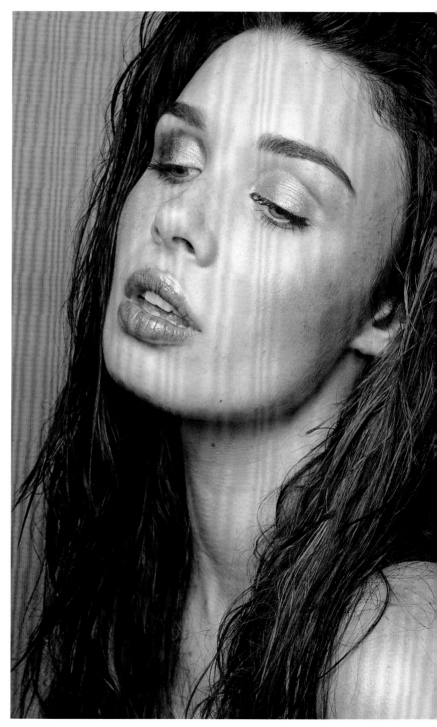

Freckles are fierce

I love freckles. I think they are just so beautiful. It makes me really sad when I see women and girls covering them with heavy make-up. However, I don't have freckles so that's easy for me to say. I suppose it's kind of like me wanting tight curly hair, and my curly-haired friends telling me I shouldn't! We are all individual and love and hate different things about our appearances. The great thing about make-up is that we can cover and add whatever we please. This look may not be for you, but for all my non-freckled friends, here's how to add a few of your own.

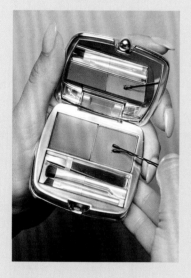

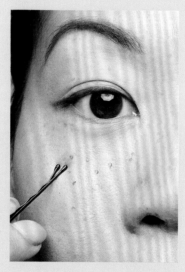

all you need...

brown eye shadow
or brow powder

a bobby pin

a cotton bud/swab

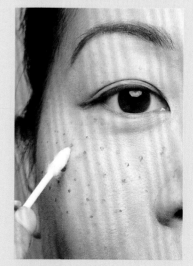

step 1 Take a soft, brown shadow. (I love using brow powders or creams as I find they last for longer on the skin.) Dip a bobby pin (yep, the ones that usually go in your hair), into the powder. This will help you create uniform freckles.

step 2 Gently tap the powdered bobby pin onto your face. Focus on the centre strip, moving from the cheek bones and across the nose. Apply as many as you like.

step 3 Using a cotton bud/swab, tap the freckles to soften them, giving them a more natural finish. Freckles complete!

Top tip

If you are a freckled beauty and want to embrace them, mixing a golden highlighter with a tinted moisturizer is the ultimate base.

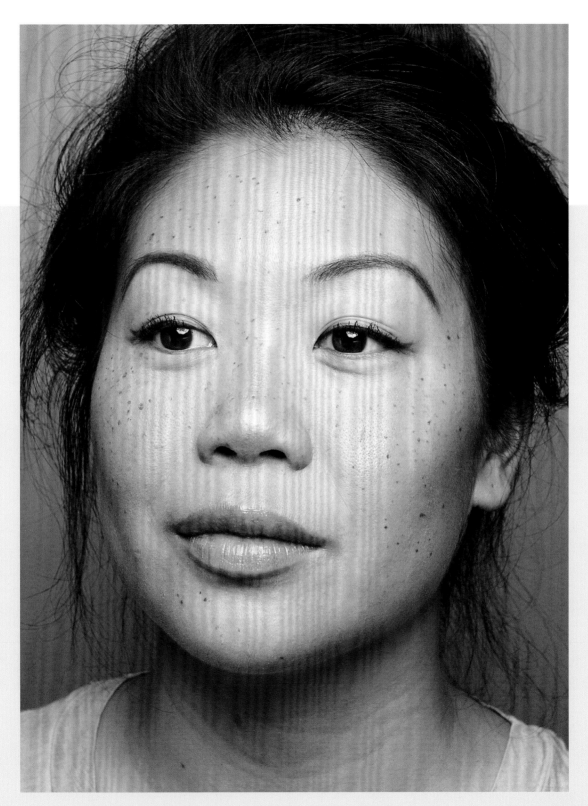

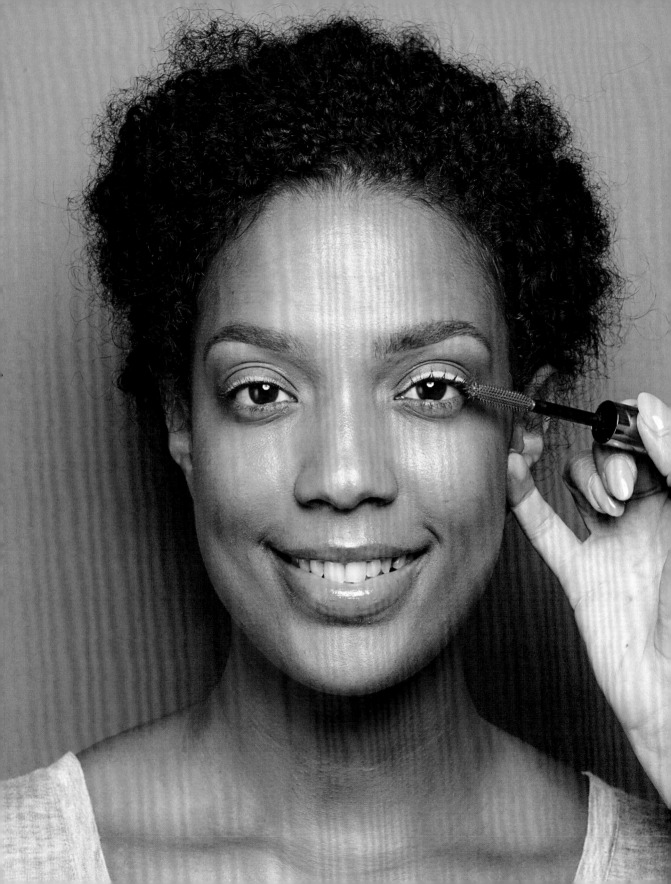

The eyes have it

Lots of make-up looks focus on the eyes and you can be really playful here.

In this chapter, I start by explaining a few basics. It's important to know which type of eyes you have so you know where to add colour and which looks to try (although, I always encourage you to try every look because each one can be adapted to suit each eye shape). So whether you have almond, downturned, round, hooded or Asian eyes, you'll know exactly what to do with liner, eye shadow, glitter and more.

I've also included a handy list of hints and tips for glasses wearers. I have worn glasses since I was 16 years old and I never let that stop me from experimenting with eye make-up so why should it stop you?!

Eye shapes

Let's talk about eye shapes. All our eyes are different but there are five main shapes and one should be similar to yours. Here, the illustrations show each shape, alongside my make-up tips for each type.

The hooded eye

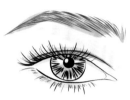

Okay, I'm starting with this one because how to apply eyeshadow for hooded eyes is one of my most requested tutorials. There are more make-up tricks for this shape than the others. It's a slightly trickier shape for applying make up, but if you follow these tips you'll have the perfect smokey eye and liner flick in no time.

✱ Apply your eye make-up with your eyes open. It's hard to see the natural crease when closed and this will help.

✱ Apply eyeshadow just above the natural crease. If you don't do this you may not be able to see the shadow at all. Make sure you buff the shadow with a clean fluffy eyeshadow brush so that the edges aren't harsh.

✱ Use an eye primer. This will help your shadow stay in place and stop it from creasing quite as much.

✱ Choose matte powder if you're unsure what to use – these are less likely to crease than shimmery ones.

✱ Curl your upper lashes to open your eyes.

✱ Wear long-wear or waterproof mascara as this is less likely to crease.

✱ Define and groom your brows. Making sure you have a good arch will lift the look of the eye.

✱ Eyeliner can be a challenge for a hooded eye. Start by drawing the line along the lash line like normal, but for the flick, keep your eye open and draw the flick from the corner of the eye up to the angle of where the brow ends. Gently pull the skin taut at your temple before extending the flick further.

The Asian eye

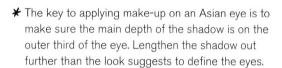

Asian eyes look amazing with an elongated eyeshadow look, such as the Bronze Shadow on pages 106–109. Eyeliner also looks fab, as you'll see on my gorgeous friend, Nicky, who modelled the Soft Flick on pages 90–93.

✱ The key to applying make-up on an Asian eye is to make sure the main depth of the shadow is on the outer third of the eye. Lengthen the shadow out further than the look suggests to define the eyes.

✱ For a quick eye look, reverse your smokey eye. By this I mean apply the darker shade near the lash line and a light shade on the rest of the eye. Blended Liner on page 98 is a similar idea.

✱ The Cut Crease on page 110–113 also looks fab on this eye shape. Particularly so because the make-up is applied in the socket for definition.

✱ Using a white liner in the waterline of the eyes will make the eyes look bigger.

✱ Try using contrasting colours of liner on the eye. A darker tone on the upper lid and a lighter shade on the lower. If you're feeling brave, apply a purple liner on the upper lid with a gold liner on the lower waterline or under the lower lash line – this colour combination looks amazing.

✱ Curl your upper lashes or use a lash-curling mascara. Apply mascara to the upper lashes only to keep the eyes looking wide.

Downturned eyes

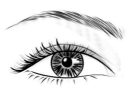

Downturned eyes tend to have a classic almond shape with plenty of room on the lid. The key is to lift the outer corner of the eye through the illusion of make-up. Here's how.

✶ Try the Classic Flick on pages 86–89, but end the line where your lashes naturally end rather than the end of the eye, then flick up. This will lift the eye.

✶ Really flick out your outer corner lashes with mascara. Tiny false lashes applied to the outer corner also look fab.

✶ Try using brown mascara on the bottom lashes and black mascara on the top to draw attention to the top of the eyes.

✶ Highlighting the centre of the eyelid with a shimmer eyeshadow will brighten the eyes. Use your ring finger to pat the product onto the lid.

✶ Avoid lining the lower waterline because this will close the eye.

✶ Don't take your eyeshadow any further out than the corner of the eye and the corner of the brow. Doing this will only add more weight to the eye.

Round eyes

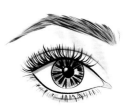

Round eyes can look really cutesy. This is lovely, but sometimes you want to look more sultry. Here are a few hints and tips.

✶ Line the upper lid from the outer corner of the eye to the inner corner of the eye with a matte black liner. This will enhance the eye shape. Flick at the end if you want to lift the eyes.

✶ Avoid lining the lower waterline. This will make the eyes too round.

✶ Smoke up the eye to counteract the cute. See pages 101–105.

✶ Apply two layers of mascara to the upper lashes and one layer to the lower lashes to make the eyes look less round.

Almond eyes

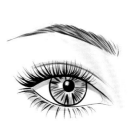

Almond eyes are the most symmetrical of eye shapes meaning they can hold pretty much any make-up look. The key is…

✶ Layer and buff your eyeshadow to perfection. Go into the socket but not further. By just going into the socket (like I do in all of the make up looks in this book), you'll hold the shape of the eye.

✶ The Classic Flick on pages 86–89 complements the almond eye beautifully.

✶ Play! You can get away with any look, so don't be afraid to experiment.

Top tip

Practice makes perfect when it comes to eye make-up. Knowing your eye shape and having the right brushes (see pages 67–68) will really help.

Eye colours

I always encourage people to play with make-up and try all different colours and shades. If it doesn't work, just wash it off! Make-up is all about experimenting and having fun. But it is also about making the most of your natural features and certain colours enhance others. So here, I have marked the most common eye colours next to the shades that will make your eyes pop. This doesn't mean you can't try other colours, in fact, you must!

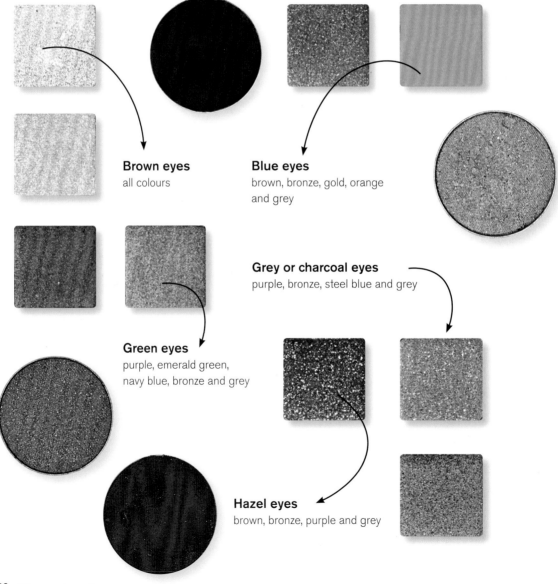

Brown eyes
all colours

Blue eyes
brown, bronze, gold, orange and grey

Grey or charcoal eyes
purple, bronze, steel blue and grey

Green eyes
purple, emerald green, navy blue, bronze and grey

Hazel eyes
brown, bronze, purple and grey

Glasses wearers

I've worn glasses and contact lenses since I was 16 years old. And on a night out I tend to sway towards wearing my contacts. But I still want my make-up to look nice when I wear my glasses. So here are my top tips for my fellow spectacle wearers.

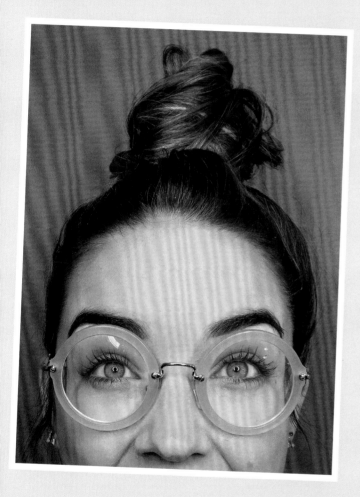

✳ Smooth skin, brighten under the eyes and the eyes themselves to counteract the shadowing from your glasses. Use a concealer two shades lighter than your skin tone. A pinky white or nude liner in the waterline also brightens the eyes.

✳ Avoid applying too much make-up around the areas that your glasses sit (the nose and the lower rim). The frame will just mark the make-up anyway and the make-up will make your glasses dirty.

✳ Eyeliner is great for glasses wearers as it defines your eyes. If you have thick frames, go for a thicker line, and if you have thin frames, go for a thinner line to match your glasses and balance your overall look.

✳ Contrast your eyeshadow with your glasses colour (i.e.: if you have purple frames go for a bronze eye rather than a purple one as this will make your eyes stand out).

✳ If your sight is as bad as mine, then it's pretty hard to even apply your make-up without contact lenses in, so use a magnifying mirror. These are great! I love the ones that light up too!

✳ Curl your upper lashes and wear a long-wear mascara so that your lashes are less likely to rub against your glasses and smear them.

✳ Make sure your eyebrows are always groomed, particularly if your glasses sit below them.

✳ Bold lipstick looks great on glasses-wearers. In opposition to what I said about eyeshadow, I actually love matching my lipstick to my frames!

Lash it up!

Before we move on to the eye looks, I wanted to share a few of my tips with you about mascara and false lashes. Some of you may be confident with this, some of you may not. Either way, I hope to help.

Applying mascara

The saying, 'Every woman should have a man that ruins their lipstick, not their mascara' is SO TRUE! Mainly because panda eyes are so hard to remove – ha! Seriously though, mascara is GREAT! It opens and defines your eyes and a good mascara can make the shortest of lashes look long and fluttery. This is the way I like to apply it.

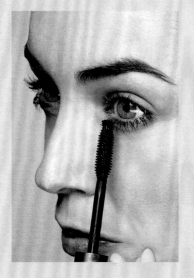

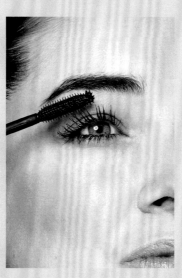

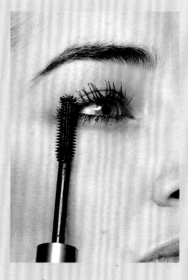

step 1 Start with the lower lashes. Yes, that's right, the lower lashes. Think about it – when you apply mascara to your lower lashes, you look up and if you already have mascara on your upper lashes and it's still a bit wet, it will transfer to your eyelids. If you're wearing eyeshadow, this can be VERY annoying and very hard to remove without ruining your look. So always, always lower lashes first!

step 2 Upper lashes next. Take your time and wiggle the brush at the roots for extra lift.

step 3 Turn the wand vertically and fan out the inner and outer corner lashes. The longer and more fanned out these tiny lashes are, the bigger your eyes will look.

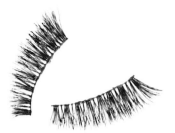

False eyelashes

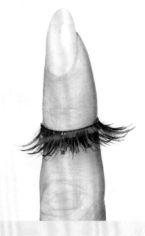

False eyelashes look amazing and can really complete a look, but they can be a little intimidating if you don't wear them regularly. Never fear, I'm here to explain how to put them on with ease so you can finish off a look with thicker, longer looking lashes and bright, wide eyes. Remember to put them on at the very end, after you have applied all of your other make-up.

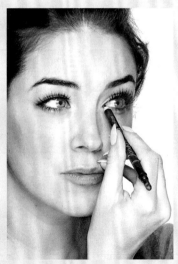

step 1 Measure each lash against your eye and trim from the inner corner to the same lenth as your lash line. Bend the lash around your finger and hold for 30 seconds to add curvature so that it sits better on your eye.

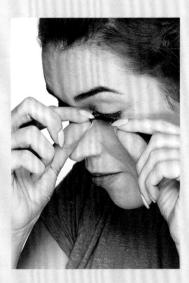

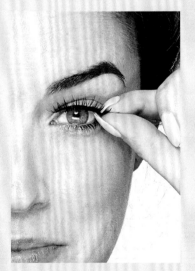

step 2 Add glue to the lash along the line with a little extra on the ends – less is more here. Wait 30 seconds for the glue to become tacky and with a mirror flat on the table, look down into it and apply the lash as close as possible to your lash line.

step 3 Squeeze the false lash and your natural lash together with your fingers to avoid a horrible gap between the two.

step 4 Finally, for a seamless finish, add black eyeliner to the gap between the inner corner of your eye and the false lash.

Get in line

I teach you about different liner looks later in the book. But I often talk about the 'waterline', so I wanted to explain what I mean by this. The waterline is the part of your eye under your top lashes and above your lower lashes and this technique is all about applying liner in the waterline.

Applying eye liner in the waterline

If you have sensitive eyes, I would avoid lining this part of the eye. If not, then give it a go. The darker the liner you use the more defined your eyes will look. If you want to brighten the eyes, use a pinky white or a nude eyeliner, as opposite. You can also line the top waterline if you want your lashes to look thicker. This can feel a bit weird to do, but looks amazing.

all you need...

waterproof kohl eyeliner

mascara

cotton bud/swab

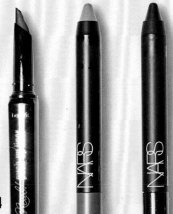

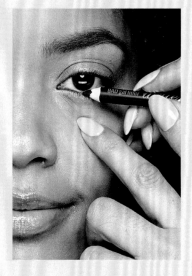

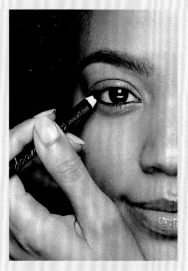

step 1 Take a sharp, waterproof kohl eyeliner and gently pull the skin beneath your lower lid to reveal the pink skin of the bottom waterline. Look straight in the mirror and apply the liner from one end to the other. Keep a cotton bud/swab to hand to dab away tears.

step 2 If you have sparse or fine lashes, line the top waterline too. Look down and gently pull your top lashes outwards to reveal the pink skin of the top waterline. Draw a line as you would the bottom waterline and repeat for depth of colour.

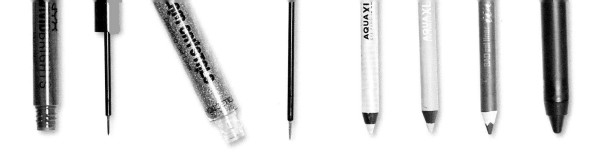

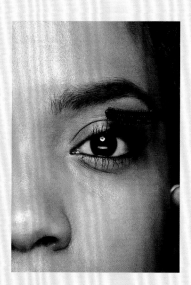

step 3 Apply mascara (see page 82) and voilà!

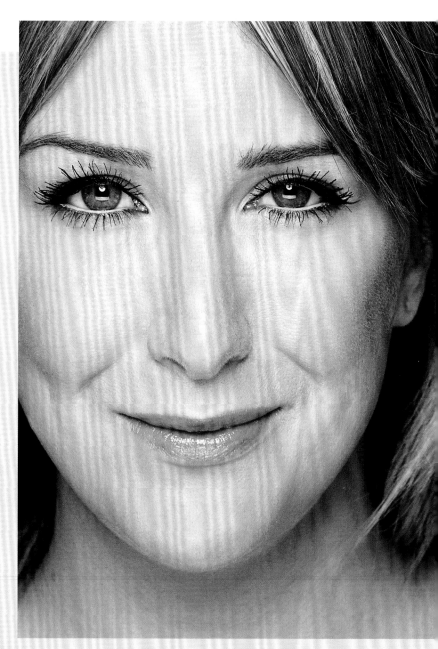

Top tip

Choose a white or nude eyeliner to line the bottom waterline if you want to open the eyes.

Classic flick

May the wings of your eyeliner always be even...

Ahh, the classic liner flick. Better known as the 'I've got one perfect eye but the other one is another story' look! Yep, we've all been there, but I have a solution, and it begins with brow mapping, that's right, you start with your brows. If your brows are mapped to perfection (see pages 40–41) then your liner will look even, I promise. Let's go!

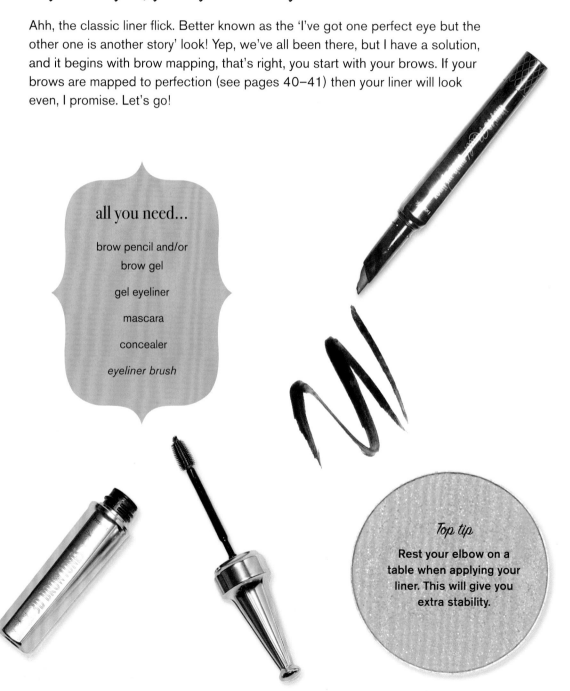

all you need...

brow pencil and/or
brow gel

gel eyeliner

mascara

concealer

eyeliner brush

Top tip

Rest your elbow on a table when applying your liner. This will give you extra stability.

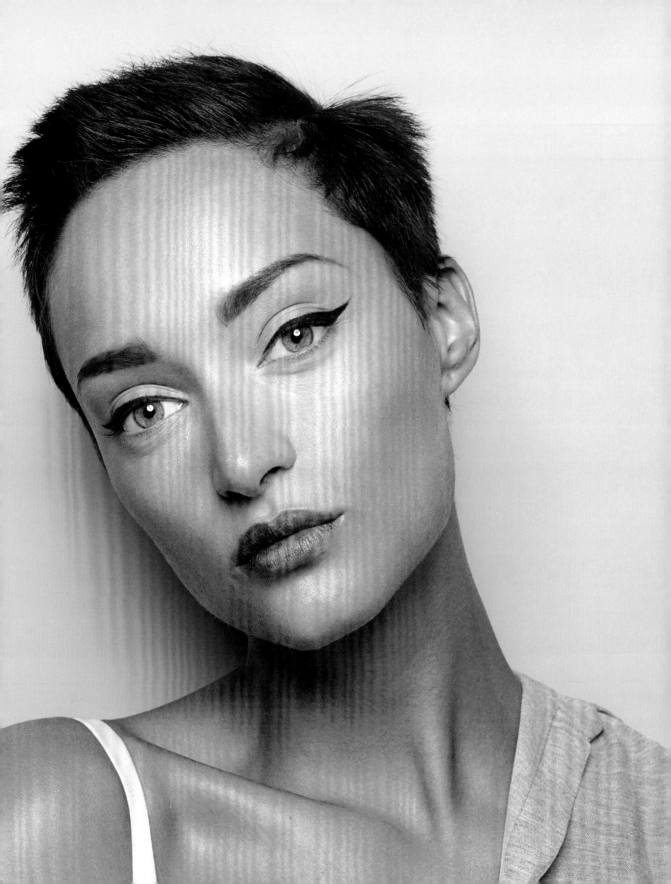

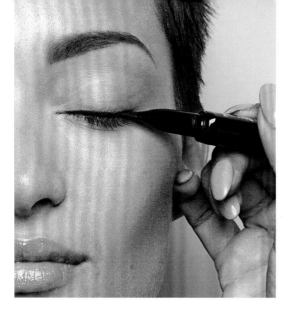

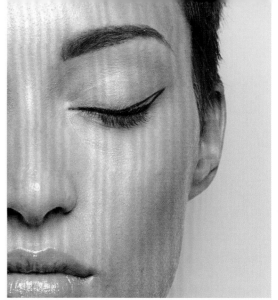

step 1 Map your brows and fill them in accordingly. Line the entire length of the lash line with your chosen eyeliner. I heart gel liners for this look as I find they are smoother to use and give a more defined finish.

step 2 (This is where the brow comes in.) Draw the line up from the outer corner of the eye up to the angle of where the brow ends. The longer the line, the bigger the flick.

step 3 Draw a line from the tip of the last line back towards the lash line. I like to swoop It back in about a third of the way along the eye.

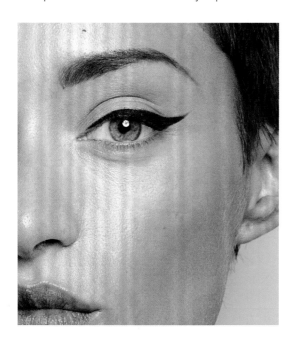

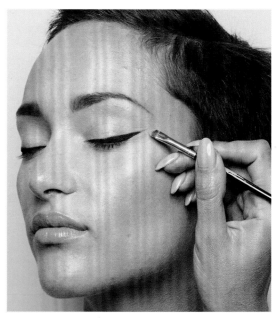

step 4 Fill in the triangular shape you have created, then add lashings of mascara (see page 82).

step 5 To sharpen the flick and to cover any mistakes, line around the eyeliner with a touch of concealer using an eyeliner brush. Repeat steps 1–5 on the other eye for even, precise flicks.

The classic liner look has been around for decades. It gives a clean, elegant finish when worn alone or with a smokey eye.

Soft flick

Sometimes in life, we just don't have time for a Classic Flick (see pages 86–89).
No matter how foolproof my technique may be, it still takes a bit of time and practise.
The soft flick on the other hand is much simpler. It is also a great starting point if you've
always struggled with eyeliner. Mainly because you use a kohl eyeliner for this look and
kohls are much softer than gel or felt-pen liners. You can blend away mistakes more easily
and the liner will still look pretty beautiful even if slightly smudged.

If you don't fancy a flick, or if your eyes don't allow for
it, then try the Blended Liner on pages 98–99.

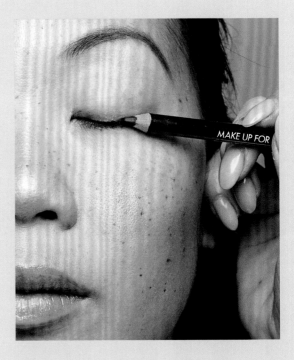

all you need...

brow pencil and/or brow gel

kohl eyeliner

eye make-up remover (optional)

mascara

glitter liquid eye liner (optional)

hard-angle brush

step 1 As with the Classic Flick, start by mapping
and defining your brows. This will still help with
drawing the angle of the flick. Draw a line along the
lash line – get as close to the lashes as possible.
Don't panic if the line is a little wonky, we will blend
it in a minute anyway.

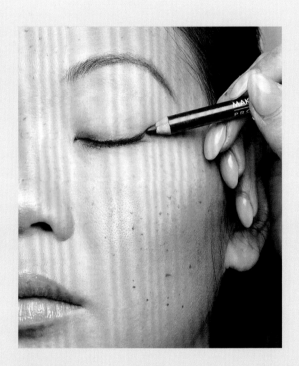

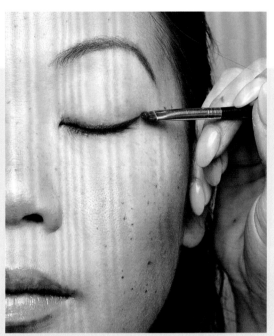

step 2 Make sure your pencil is sharp and draw a flick from the lash line at the corner of the eye at the angle towards the tail of the brow. (You don't need to swoop back in with this look, just draw the line.)

step 3 Now for the magic. Take a hard-angled eyeshadow brush (it must be hard angled as this is going to create the definition and shape). Start by going over the line along the lash line with the brush to soften it and blend it into shape. Then lightly draw over the flick. Only brush upwards on the flick – don't go backwards and forwards with the brush here. This will create a more defined shape. (If you want an even sharper flick, clean the brush and dip it in a touch of make-up remover. Draw around the flick with the eye make-up remover to remove any excess liner. Then add mascara (see page 82).

See finished look overleaf.

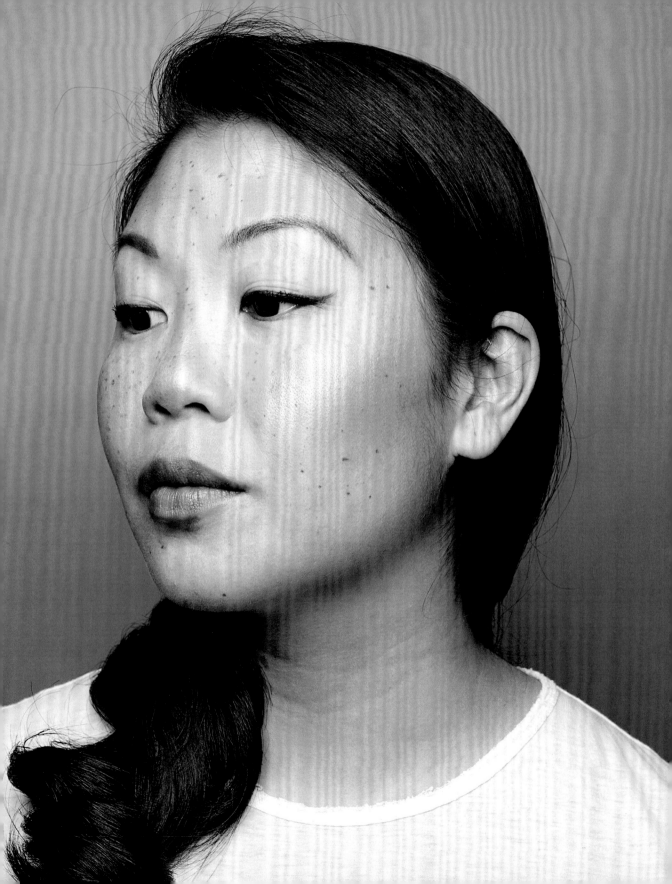

I love this look as there are so many different coloured kohl pencils out there. And this is a great way to experiment with colour. I also love the liners that have a touch of sparkle in them. So experiment and have fun with this look.

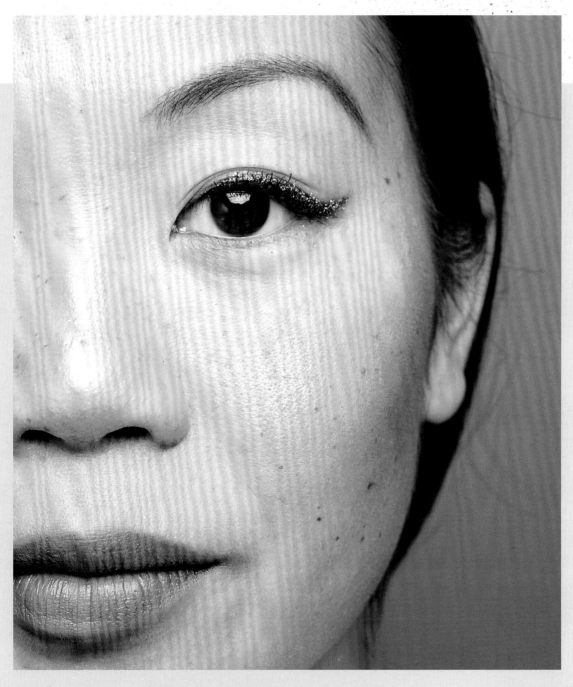

Bright liner and lashes

Blue mascara is my thing. I rock it most days. No, I don't have an obsession with the 80s, but I do have an obsession with brighter, whiter looking eyes. And that's exactly what blue mascara does. In fact, coloured mascara is a bit of a gem in the make-up world. It's bold enough to wear alone, and can boost the look of your eye colour with one sweep. Keep the skin dewy and the lips nude to make it all about the eyes. Add coloured liner if you feel confident. Try any colour you like but to really complement your eye colour, try these shades…

Green eyes blue and violet

Blue eyes browns, bright blues and purples

Brown eyes any colour!

Hazel eyes greens and golds

Grey or charcoal eyes steel blue and purple

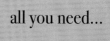

all you need...

kohl eyeliner in any colour you like

mascara in any colour you like

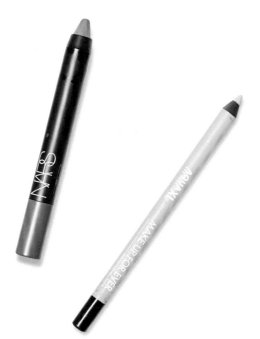

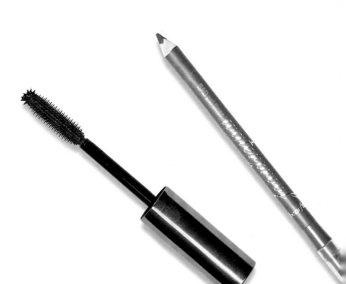

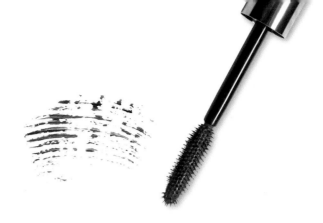

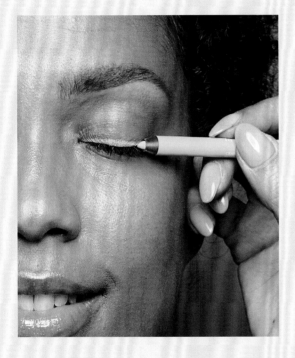

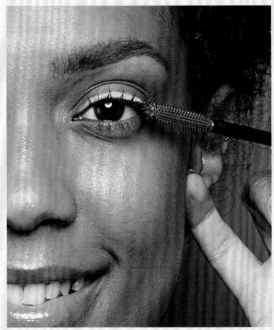

step 1 Line the lash line with your chosen eyeliner. Keep the line simple. No flick required.

step 2 Layer on your coloured mascara of choice (see page 82).

Look how great this look is using purple liner and blue mascara opposite!

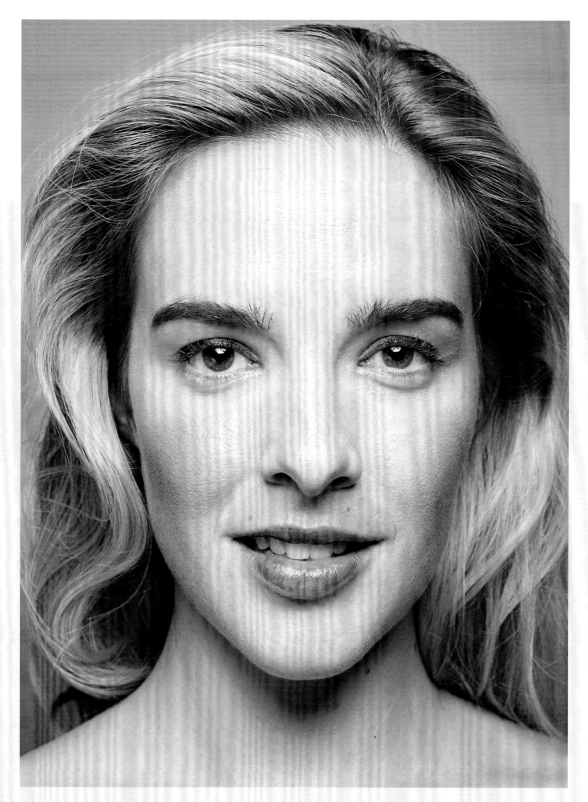

Blended liner

One question I get asked a lot, particularly by older women, is, 'How can I enhance my eyes?' There are a few answers out there, one of them being groomed, defined brows. You can read all about that on pages 36–53.

But a soft line of shadow or liner on the upper lid can also help to add definition. This is also a great quick-fix make-up look for when you're in a rush, as well as being a great introductory look if you're a make-up newbie. Pair it with a dewy base and and any lip colour you like.

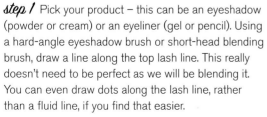

all you need...

powder or cream eyeshadow, or gel or kohl eyeliner

mascara

hard-angle or short-head blending brush

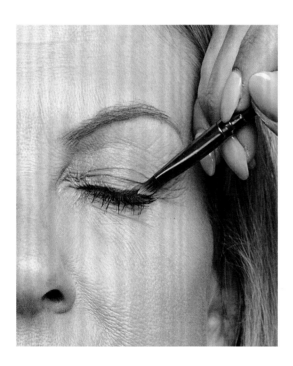

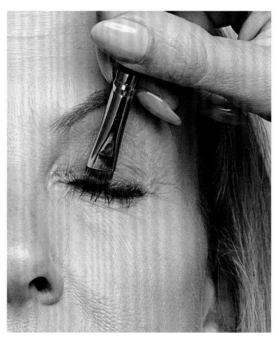

step 1 Pick your product – this can be an eyeshadow (powder or cream) or an eyeliner (gel or pencil). Using a hard-angle eyeshadow brush or short-head blending brush, draw a line along the top lash line. This really doesn't need to be perfect as we will be blending it. You can even draw dots along the lash line, rather than a fluid line, if you find that easier.

step 2 Hold your brush vertically (like I am in the picture) and blend the line upwards. You can do this as much or as little as you like. If you want it to be really smokey, you can always add a matching powder eyeshadow over the top of the line (or more eyeshadow if that is your choosen product), then blend, blend, blend.

Finish with mascara and a smile on your face, in the knowledge that you have defined your eyes in a matter of minutes!

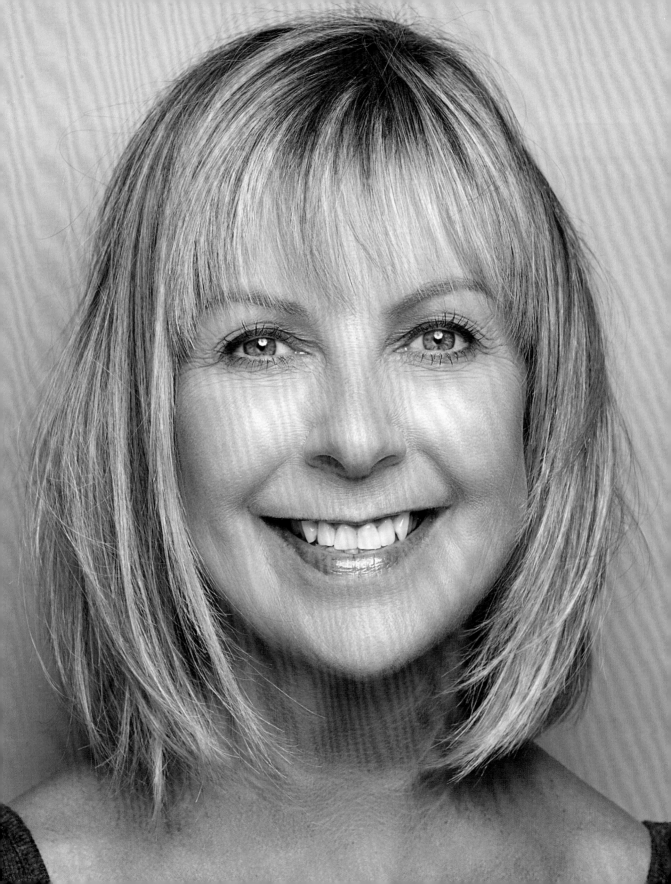

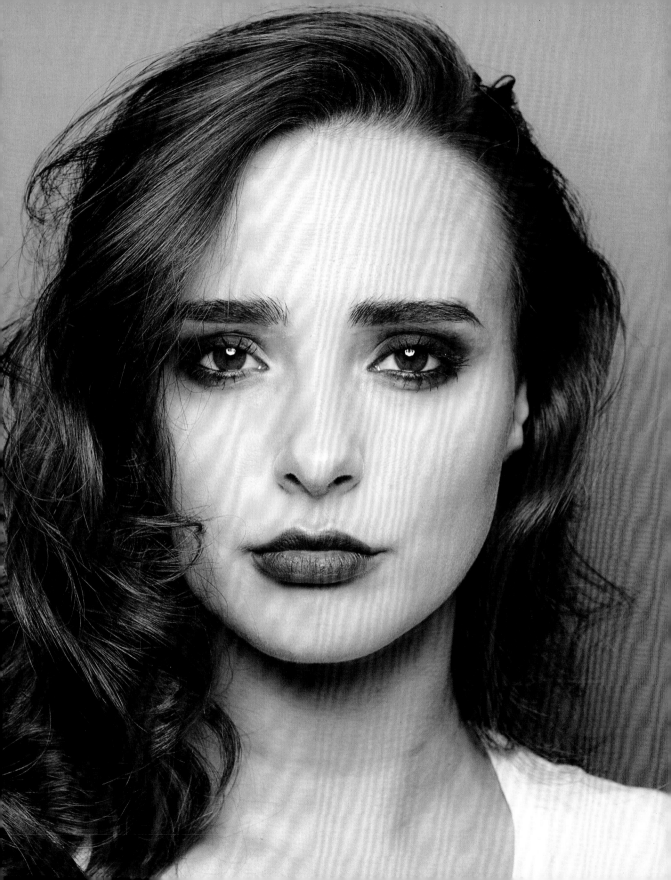

Classic smokey eye

The classic smokey eye is a dreamy thing. When done properly is can look both elegant and sultry all wrapped into one gorgeous look! I love using matte greys and blacks for the ultimate version but you can choose other colours and follow the same technique. Pair it with a nude lip for the ultimate sophistication. Or vamp it up with a stained berry lip by layering a lip stain on your lips followed by patting a lipstick over the top with your ring finger. Whether you choose to rock this look with jeans and a T-shirt or with a little black dress, remember, you look great!

A softer version of this look works beautifully on an older eye. Avoid steps 6–8 to keep the look elegant and fresh, and smoke away.

all you need...

eye primer

4 x eyeshadows in gradient colour (I use vanilla, soft taupe, light grey and black)

black gel eyeliner

black kohl eyeliner

mascara

fluffy eyeshadow brush

pencil brush

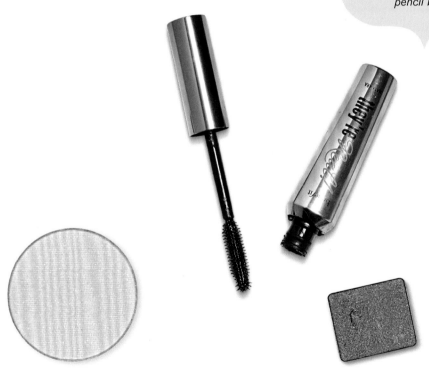

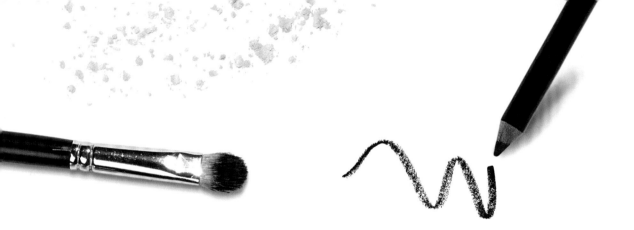

step 1 Prime your eyes. Eye primers are great. They keep your eye make-up in place, enhance the pigment of the shadow and prevent it from creasing.

step 2 Buff a vanilla shade eyeshadow over your eyelid. (This is your base shadow.)

step 3 Contour the eye socket with a soft taupe eyeshadow. This isn't a step that many people are used to doing. But it really adds a softness to the look and also helps to map out the rest of the look.

★ ★

step 4 Buff a light grey, matte eyeshadow into the socket and on the outer third of the eye.

step 5 Blend a black matte eyeshadow in the outer corner of the eye.

step 6 Line the lash line with a black gel eyeliner and then, using a touch of the black eyeshadow on a pencil brush, blend the liner up to give a soft, smokey effect.

★ ★

step 7 Line the upper and lower waterline with a black kohl pencil. Draw a small amount of the liner under the lower lash line too and blend back and forth with the pencil brush to create an under smoke beneath the eye.

step 8 Blend the matte grey shadow used in step 4 under the lower lash line and over the liner to bring the look together

step 9 Sweep on tonnes of black mascara (bottom lashes first so that you don't transfer mascara to the eyelid when you look up to do the bottom lashes). Clean under the eyes, add your base, bronzer and blusher, brush up those brows and finish with your chosen lip colour.

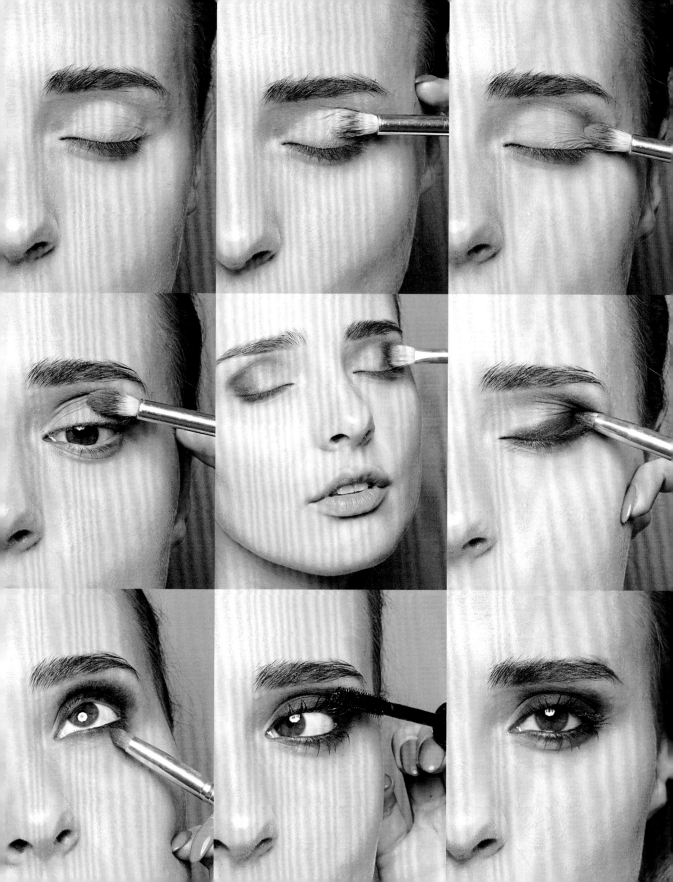

Colourful smokey eye

A colourful smokey eye is one of my favourite looks. You'll find loads of different colour options on my YouTube channel and also in my first book. I love a colourful smokey eye as it can really make an entire look. Even if you're just wearing a white shirt and black jeans, a bright eye can add elegance, glamour and an edge to your look.

The colours available are endless, so I suggest picking colours that you love the look of (or that match your new shoes)! Just have fun – remember, it's only make-up! A good thing to remember is that rich, jewel-toned shadows, like the green used here, tend to suit everyone. Try different textures too – I use creams and powders to add a different dimension to the look.

all you need...

brow pencil and/or brow gel

eye primer

4 x eyeshadows

black gel eyeliner

black kohl eyeliner

mascara

fluffy eyeshadow brush

pencil brush or cotton bud/swab

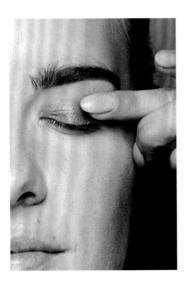 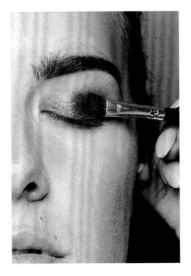 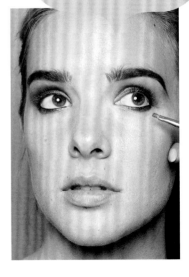

step 1 Define the brows (I love the Feathered Brow on pages 52–53 with this look). Prime the eyes and pat a cream eyeshadow in your chosen colour all over the eyelid and up to the socket of the eye. When using a cream shadow, I like to use my fingers as I find the warmth helps blend into the skin.

step 2 Using a fluffy eyeshadow brush, gently blend a matching metallic eyeshadow over the top of the cream. Focusing mainly on the centre of the eye – the metallic finish of the shadow will highlight the eye.

step 3 Line the lower waterline with a black kohl eyeliner, then blend the cream eyeshadow used in step 1 under the lower lash line, around three-quarters of the way towards the inner eye. Layer the metallic shadow over the top of this and blend the two together using a pencil brush or cotton bud/swab. Take care not to blend the cream shadow too close to the inner corner of the eye. Keep the highlighting metallic shadow on the inner corner to brighten the look.

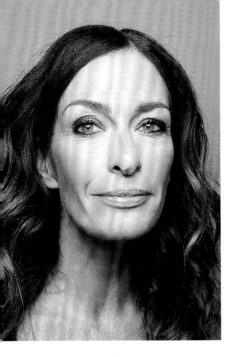

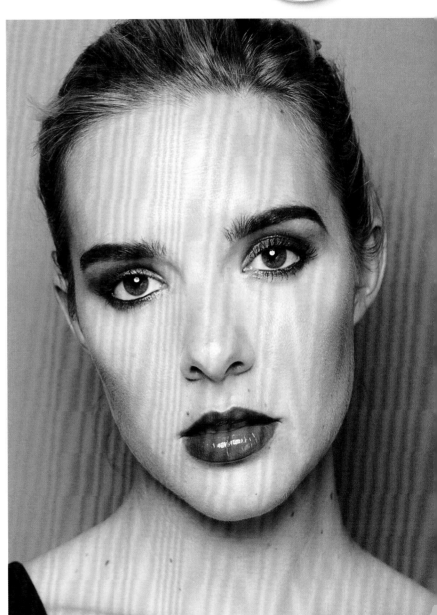

Don't be afraid to try a colourful smokey eye if you are a little older. See what colours suit your eye shade on page 80.

step 4 Add tonnes of black mascara. Apply your base, then add your chosen lip colour. I personally think this look works with a nude or a berry-red, glossy lip.

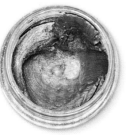

Bronze shadow

I've said it before and I'll say it again, bronze shadows are the queens of eyeshadows. Mainly because they suit everyone, whatever you age, skin tone or eye colour. There are so many different shades and finishes in the bronze category. So your best bet is to buy an eyeshadow palette. These include shadows that work well together, meaning some of the job is done for you! This bronze look is beautiful for a night out, a shopping day or even a wedding! You can always play it down by not including the liner in the waterline. Or play it up by going for deeper bronzer.

all you need...

eye primer

3 x eyeshadows (I use nude, matte brown, deep bronze)

copper or gold metallic eyeshadow

black gel liner or black eyeshadow

mascara

black kohl pencil

fluffly eyeshadow brush

lip brush

blending brush

Top tip

Define your brows before you begin the steps. Your brows balance your face. This will help you to know how much shadow to add.

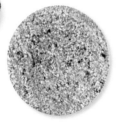

Top tip

Apply your eye make-up before your base. Eyeshadow will more than likely fall under the eyes when you're blending, so by doing the eyes first, you can just wipe away any excess shadow without ruining your base.

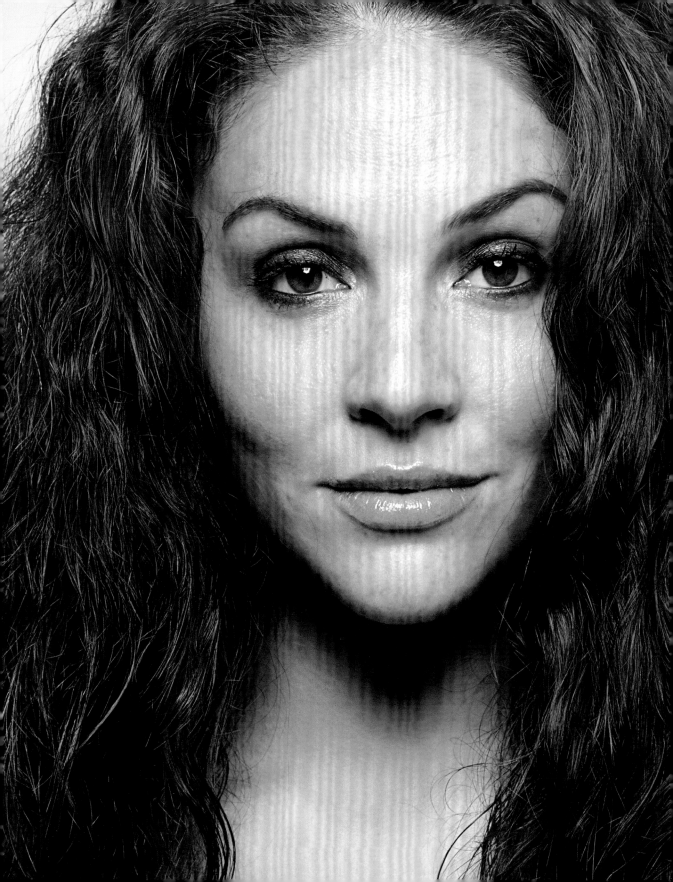

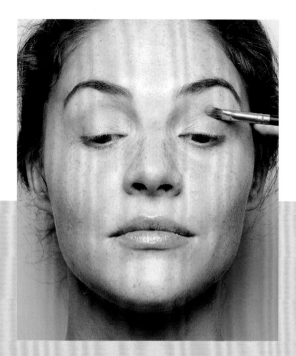

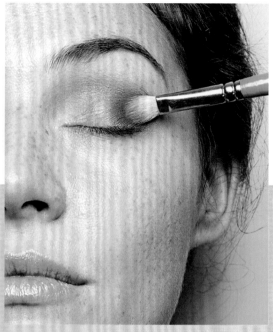

step 1 Prime the eyes and set with a nude eyeshadow. This will create the perfect, no-crease base, ready for layering different textured shadows. Contour the socket of the eye with a matte brown eyeshadow (I actually used a bronzer for this.)

step 2 Using a fluffy eyeshadow brush, blend a deep bronze shadow into the socket of the eye and around the outer third of the eyelid to smoke up the look.

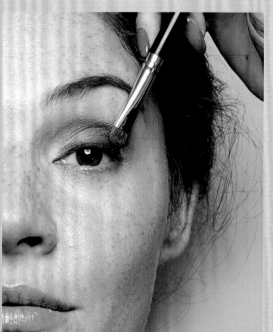

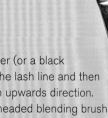

step 3 Take a gel black liner (or a black eyeshadow), apply this on the lash line and then smudge along the line in an upwards direction. Use a hard-angle or short-headed blending brush for this as the small head means I have full control when blending. This will define the eye.

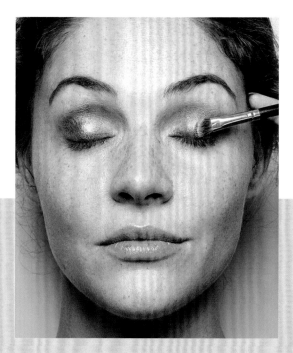

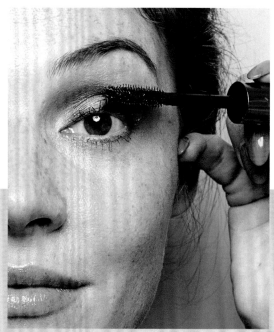

step 4 Press a copper or gold, metallic eyeshadow into the centre of the lid to highlight the high point of the eyelid. Buff out the edges gently.

step 5 Apply lashings of black mascara. I add mascara now, rather than at the end, so that I can gauge how much more depth of colour the eye can take.

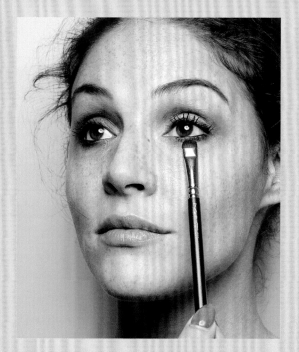

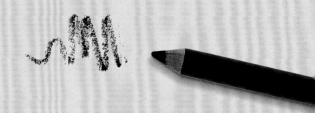

step 6 Line the inner waterlines with a kohl pencil and smudge under the lower lash line slightly. Blend a touch of the deep bronze eyeshadow from step 2 over the top to soften.

Add your base, bronzer, blusher and highlighter and pair the look with a creamy nude lip. Oh you bronzed beauty you!

If you want a really quick bronze shadow look, just buff one shade over the lid and under the lower lash line and add mascara.

The cut crease

The cut crease has become an Instagram sensation! This look is a bit more complex than a smokey eye. It works best on big, almond or round eyes. But it looks super-cool when done right. You can use any colours you like. The look itself is quite bold so I stick with neutral tones.

all you need...

eye primer

contour cream

matte taupe eyeshadow

concealer

glitter

Vaseline

gel liner

mascara

false lashes (optional)

pencil brush

hard-angle brush

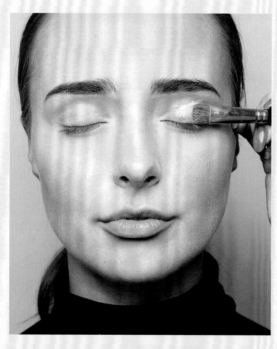

step 1 Fill in your brows and prime the entire eyelid up to the brow bone.

step 2 Keeping your eyes open, apply a contour cream into the socket of your eye and extend outwards, following the shape of the eye. This line doesn't have to be perfect. Think of it as a guideline for the rest of the look. Then take a taupe matte shadow and buff over the line with a pencil brush to soften it slightly.

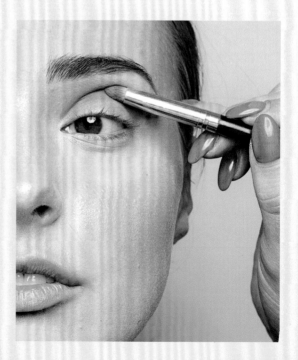

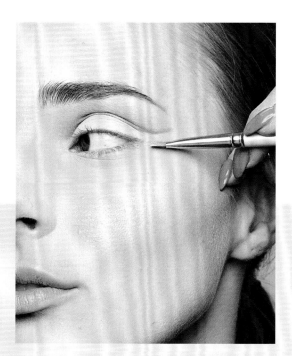

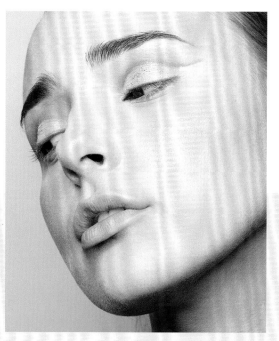

step 3 Next, take your concealer and fill in the base, up to where the line you have created begins. This will help to sharpen the look.

step 4 Take a glitter of your choice and pat over the concealer. If it's a loose glitter, use a small amount of Vaseline to stick it in place.

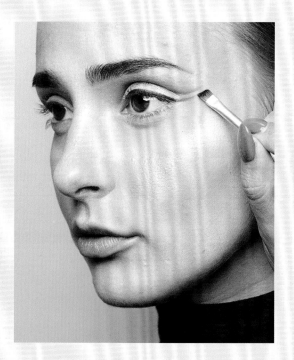

step 5 Time to wing it out. This is slightly different to the Classic Flick (see pages 86–89) because you are mirroring the shape of the crease line. Start by applying the line along the lash line, and then flick it out so it is parallel to the crease line.

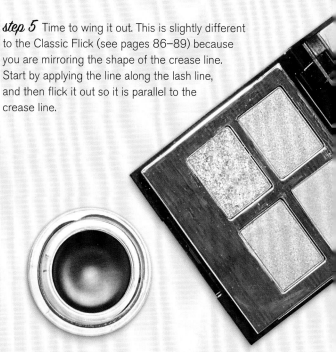

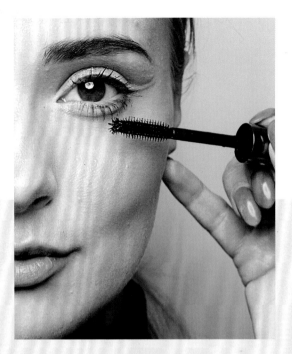

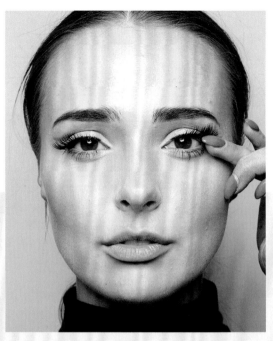

step 6 Add loads of black mascara. I love to add more than usual on the bottom lashes for this look.

step 7 For extra glamour, add some false lashes. If you do this, make sure you go back over the lash line with eyeliner to cover the band of the lashes.

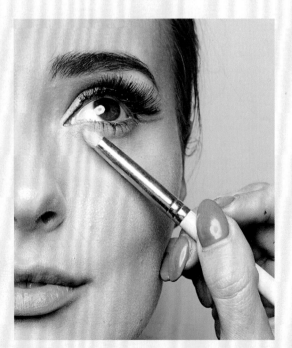

step 8 Blend the taupe eyeshadow from step 2 under your lower lash line. Then add your favourite lipstick, or stick with a nude lip. You are now most certainly 'selfie ready'!

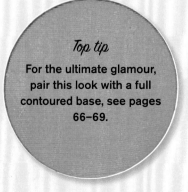

Top tip

For the ultimate glamour, pair this look with a full contoured base, see pages 66–69.

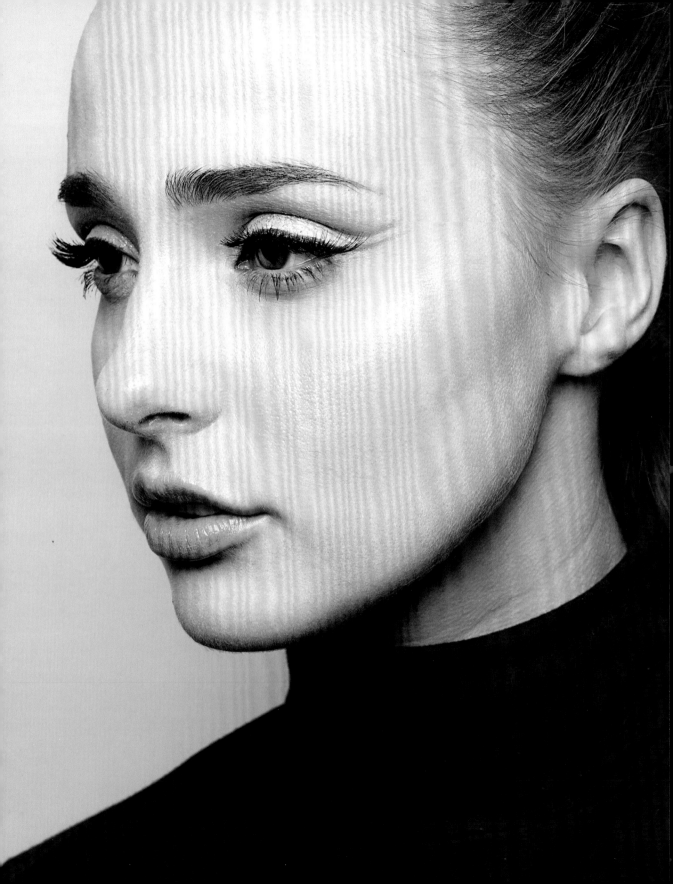

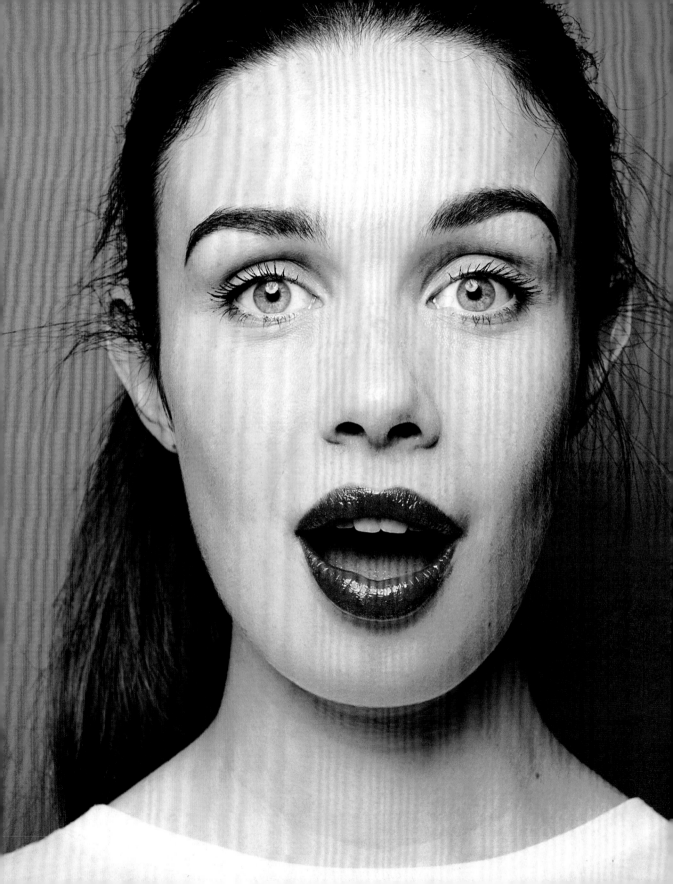

Luscious lips

Pucker up! It's time to get those lips in shape.

I love red lipstick so I've started there with the looks in this chapter. Lining the lips is key to achieving the perfect red lip but also for shaping and filling in lips if you don't naturally have the perfect cupid's bow. I explain the ways in which you can line different lip shapes to make it easy for you to create a full, kissable pout in no time.

And why stop with red (do you know that I LOVE colour, yet?) Try one or all of the other looks here for glossy, nude, matte and highlighted lips.

Lip shapes

I love lipstick, but I didn't really suit it until I'd worked out how to apply it properly. You see, I have thin lips and lipstick on thin lips can get pretty messy if it's just chucked on. Unless you have perfectly full lips, you may understand my frustration. We all come in different shapes and sizes, and our lips are no exception. If you've always wondered how to make the most of your lips, how to make them look fuller, or even thinner, how to accentuate your cupid's bow, or how to stop your lipstick from bleeding, then here's how. Let's start with the different lip shapes and where to apply your lipstick and liner to get the perfect pout.

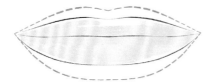

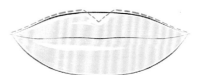

Thin lips

This is me! The key to plumping up thin lips is to over-line your lips slightly – not too much.

✱ Use a lip liner to line around the outside of your lips following the dotted lines above. Follow the natural shape of your lips so that you don't look like a cartoon!

✱ If you have a thin lower lip, draw slightly underneath the lip line and along the lip line on top to balance out your bottom lip with your top one.

✱ Filling in a thin top lip takes practice. Over-draw your top lip slightly. Going too high will look odd, so be sure to follow your natural lip shape, just above it. Try this out at home and see how you feel when you catch a glance of yourself in the mirror. Adjust the line until you are happy to show the world your beautiful self!

Oval lips

This is a great shape lip, but there tends to be no definition on the cupid's bow.

✱ Draw a cross in the centre of your upper lip (see pages 122–123), then draw out around the natural lip line. If you really want to make your cupid's bow stand out, use a lip liner slightly deeper than your natural lip colour.

✱ Fill in your lips with lipstick and revel in the beautifully bowed top lip you have created. Genius!

Top tip

It's so annoying when your lipstick runs outside your lip line. The best thing to do is to conceal around the lip line. This will act like a barrier. If you find your lipstick runs a lot, stick to a matte product as glosses move more.

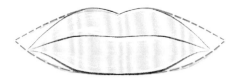

Downturned lips

This lip shape can make you look sad, so lengthen the outer corners following the dotted lines above to elongate your smile.

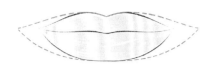

Small lips

If you have small lips, the best thing to do is to elongate them at the outer corners, up to the top of the cupid's bow. Follow the dotted line above to make lips look fuller.

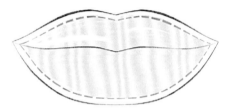

Large full lips

To make your lips look less full, draw liner on your lips, just below and above your lip line following the dotted lines above. Then conceal around the lips with the concealer you would use on your face, covering your natural lip line.

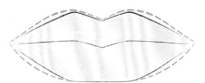

Sharp lips

Soften sharp lips by rounding off the cupids bow and the outer corners. Make sure your liner is blended in perfectly to add to the softening effect.

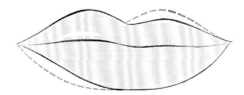

Uneven lips

Mirror the even side of your lips with your lip liner. Fill in the entire lip with the liner to create an even base before you add lipstick over the top.

Top tip

Use a nude lip liner, the same colour as your lips, to define your lips to begin with. Then fill in with your lipstick, gloss or coloured liner.

Lip products

A good lipstick can really change your whole look. If I'm feeling a bit down, or if my skin is looking a touch dull, I'll chuck on a lipstick and feel better instantly! There are so many colours to choose from, but there are four main types of product. Lip liners, lipsticks, lip stains and lip glosses. You can use them individually, all together or not at all! It really is up to you.

Lip liners

Do not skip lining your lips. Lip liners are amazing for adding definition, changing your lip shape (see pages 116–117) and for helping keep your lipstick in place for longer. Although some people find lining a bit tricky, my advice is to give it a go. My top tip is to always make sure liners are sharp and not warm. If you know you're about to create a badass bright lip, put your lip liner in the fridge for 10 minutes to make sure it's not too soft to use. If you are in a rush, but still want to define your lips, try a lipstick and liner in one. Yep, these now exist thanks to Benefit Cosmetics!

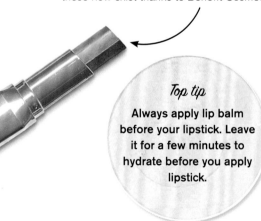

Top tip
Always apply lip balm before your lipstick. Leave it for a few minutes to hydrate before you apply lipstick.

Lipsticks

Okay, there are thousands of colours out there to choose from, like, actually thousands! Play! Don't be afraid to try different colours out. If you go to a make-up counter, don't try a lippy out on the back of your hand and hope for the best. Ask the make-up artist to sanitize it for you and then try it on your lips. You'll be surprised at how different it looks on. Choosing the texture of your lipstick is most important as it really does change the look of the lip. The three main textures are:

Matte
The formula used to create these lipsticks gives no shine at all, they are quite flat but can look great. They tend to be long-wear, but avoid them if you have dry lips as they will only accentuate the dryness.

Satin
This is the most common type. They are slightly oilier and more hydrating than matte products. This is the type of lipstick I recommend for everyday wear.

Shimmer
Remember I spoke about my fave 90s lipstick, Heather Shimmer, well yep, that was this formula. These give a lovely shimmer to the lip but can be quite ageing.

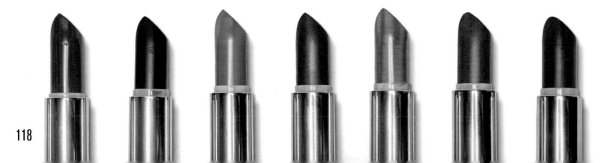

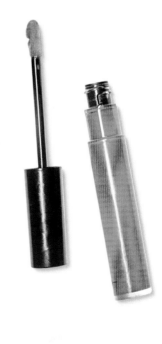

I decant my lipsticks into a palette as it's easier for me to see them and lighter for me to carry. I hate having to throw the beautiful packaging away but this technique is a make-up artist must!

Lip stains

Lip stains do exactly what they say, they stain the lip. Not forever mind you, just until you take them off. These are great for a subtle hint of colour and they are also fab underneath a lipstick as at least you know when your lipstick has worn off, your stain will still be there holding the fort until you make it to a mirror!

Lip glosses

I have a love-hate relationship with lip glosses. I love them when they make my lips look hydrated and plump. I hate them when half of the hair from my head is stuck to them! Some glosses are really thick – these are the ones that last the longest and they are also the stickiest. Thin glosses are lovely and hydrating, and tend not to be as sticky, but don't last as long. Sometimes I mix the two together for a compromise.

Top tip

If you suffer with dry lips, try a lip scrub, such as Fresh Brow Sugar Lip Scrub, Glam Glow Pout Mud Fizzy Lip Exfoliator and Lush Bubblegum Lip Scrub. Alternatively, gently exfoliate your lips with a dry toothbrush.

If red lipstick were a woman, she'd run the world!

A red lipstick is one of the most powerful pieces of make-up you can own. It adds a touch of glamour that no other make-up product can compete with. Whether you're a mum or a movie star, a red pout makes you feel like you can achieve anything. However, perfecting the application of a red lip can be a challenge. Of course you can apply it straight from the bullet, but, for many of us, that ends up in wonky looking lips and lipstick on teeth! So this is my favourite way to apply a red lipstick to ensure definition, long wear and perfection. You can, of course, use this technique with any colour you like!

all you need...

lip exfoliator

concealer

lip primer

lip liner

lipstick

gloss (optional)

tissue

2 lip brushes

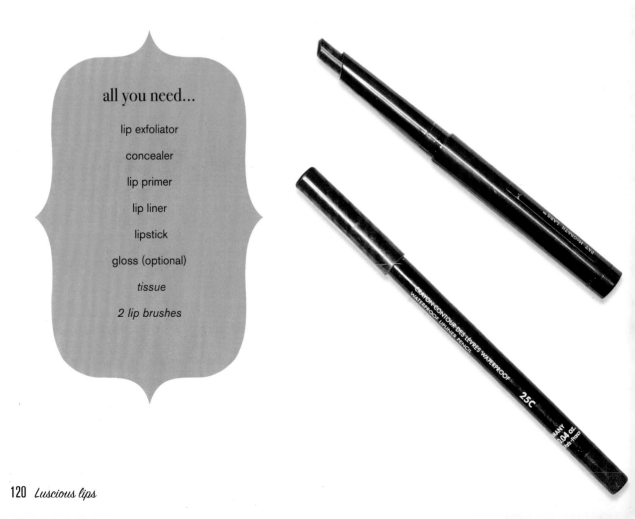

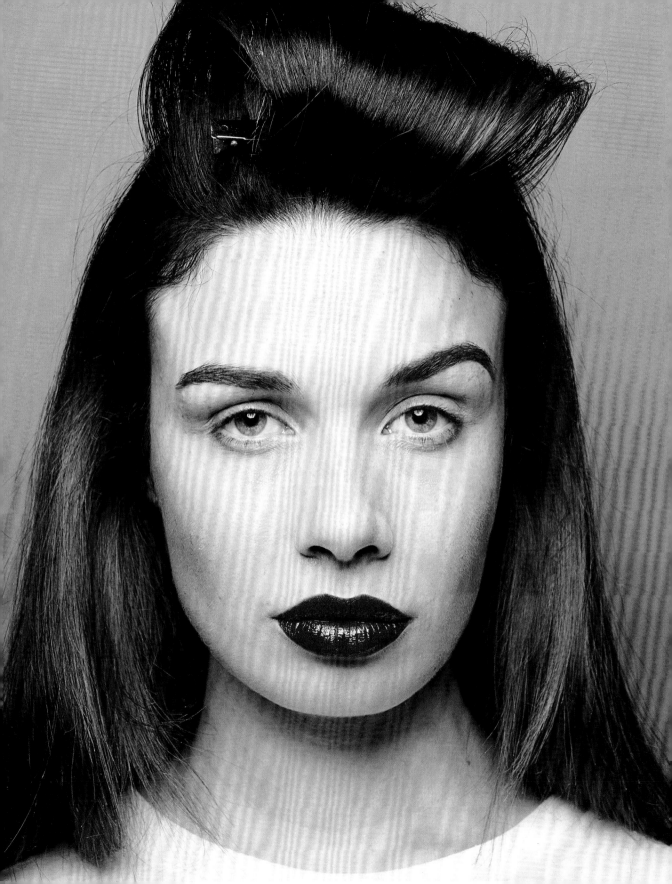

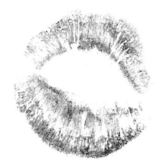

step 1 Exfoliate your lips. (I heart the Lush Bubblegum Scrub, mainly because it tastes delish!) Dry your lips with a tissue and pat a small amount of concealer all over the lips. This will help to fill in any lines, priming them ready for lipstick, and help keep your lippy in place for longer.

step 2 Using a lip liner in a similar red to your lipstick, draw a cross in the centre of your lips. This will define (or create if your lips are like mine) your cupid's bow and ultimately give you the perfect-looking pout!

step 3 Draw a line under or along the bottom of the lower lip for definition.

step 4 Draw a line down the sides of the top lip from the cross. (All of these steps will make your lips look fuller, believe me.)

step 5 Colour in the outer corners of your lips, top and bottom. This is the area that your lipstick tends to vanish from first, especially after a cocktail! By applying liner here, the colour will stay put for longer. Adding a depth of colour here and not in the centre of the lips will also create the illusion of fuller lips.

step 6 Take your lipstick and a lip brush (Karla Powell's are my favourite) and carefully apply your lipstick all over the lips.

step 7 Using a clean lip brush and concealer, draw a line around your lips for extra definition. This will also prevent the colour of your lipstick from bleeding.

step 8 Leave the lips matte or add a gloss over the top.

step 9 There you have it, perfect red lips.

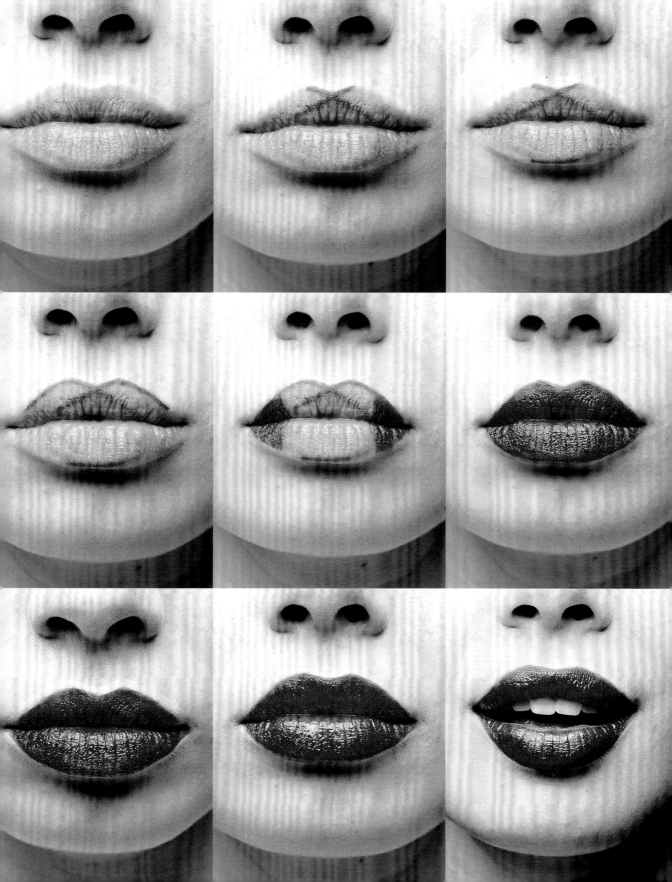

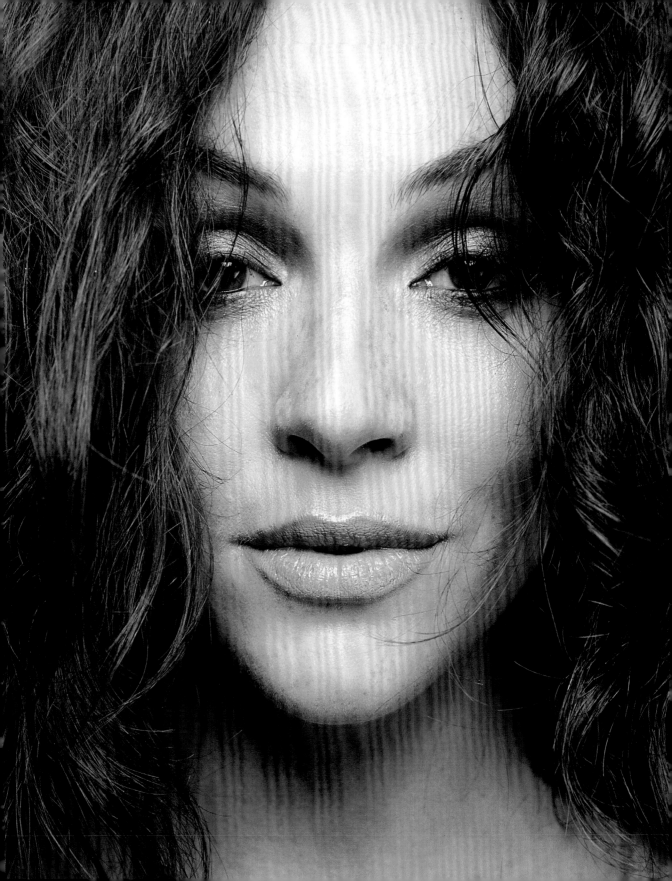

Nude lips

I love nude lips. I think this is because I have thin lips. And although a nude lip looks great on all lip shapes. It really helps make a thin lip look fuller. But, as a matter of fact, it can make any lip look fuller. It's all about the technique. When picking a nude lip, you have two options. One, pick a shade that matches your lip colour perfectly. This will give you the most natural of lip looks. Two, pick a nude lip liner and lipstick that work well together and prime your lips first – this is what I do here.

all you need...

lip primer

lip liner

lipstick

highlighter

lip brush

step 1 Prime your lips by patting either a lip primer or concealer lightly over your lips. This will knock back the redness in your lips, meaning you get the true colour of the lip products. It will also help to fill in any fine lines and keep your lipstick in place.

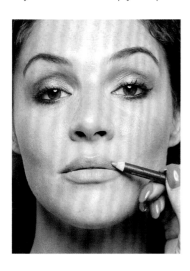

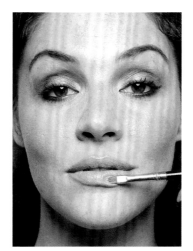

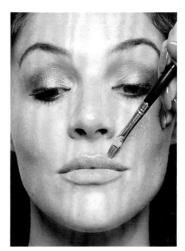

step 2 Line the lips. First, make sure the liner is sharp. Then you have three options. If you have good lips like the lovely Steph here, line the lips by following the natural lip line. If you have thinner lips, line just over the lip line. And if you want super-defined lips, follow the lip steps on pages 120–123.

step 3 Fill in your lips with your chosen lipstick. I like to use a lip brush for this as I find it gives me more precision. Using a brush also means that you can blend in the liner slightly, without losing any of the definition.

step 4 Highlight the cupid's bow of the lip with a highlighter. This will make your pout pop, make your lips look fuller and it looks awesome in pictures.

Complete. A nude lip is like that trusty old pair of denim jeans. Always there when you need it, and it goes with everything!

Running around nude!

No, I'm not talking naked nude, I'm talking nude make-up nude!
And in particular nude lipstick.

If you're in a rush and just need a quick cool look, then
take out your nude lipstick and swipe it over your eyes,
cheeks, oh, and your lips. Blend it in, brush up your
brows and well, that's it! Try this with other shades
of lipstick too if you dare. It's the one-stop shop of
make-up looks!

all you need...

nude lipstick

blending brush

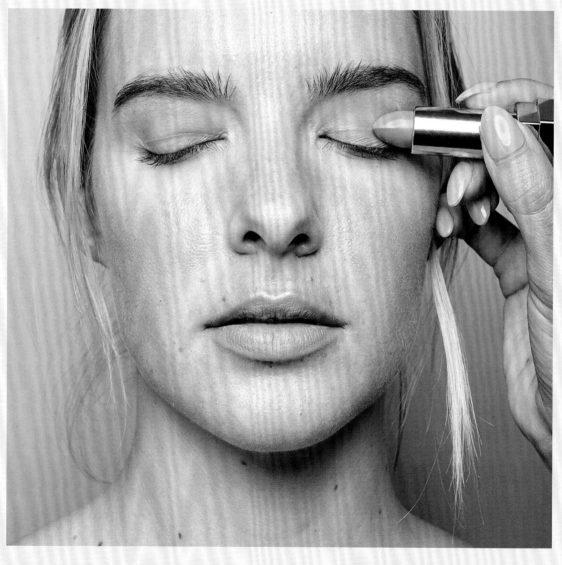

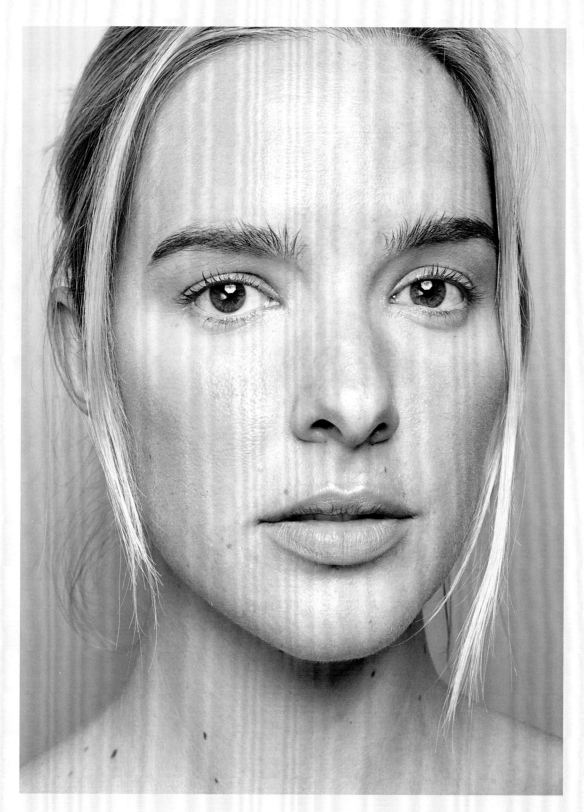

Matte lips

A matte lip looks gorgeous, especially if you pair it with a metallic eyeshadow. There are now more matte lipsticks to choose from than ever, but what if your absolute favourite lipstick doesn't come in matte? Well, I have the solution for you as there's a really quick and easy way to make any lipstick matte. Here's how…

all you need…

lip primer

lipstick

lip liner (optional)

loose translucent powder

lip brush

tissue

blusher brush

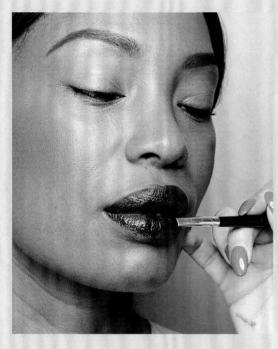

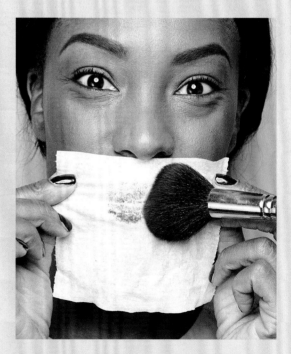

step 1 Apply your lipstick like normal. You can do this with or without a lip liner.

step 2 Take a piece of tissue (yes, a piece of tissue!) and hold it over your lips. It should be slightly touching your lips.

step 3 Take a loose, translucent powder and a blusher brush, and dust the powder over the tissue where your lips are. (Betsy had no idea what I was doing in this shot, hence her 'what is going on?' expression!) Repeat this 2–3 times. Remove the tissue and like magic, your lipstick is now matte. HOW. COOL. IS. THAT?!

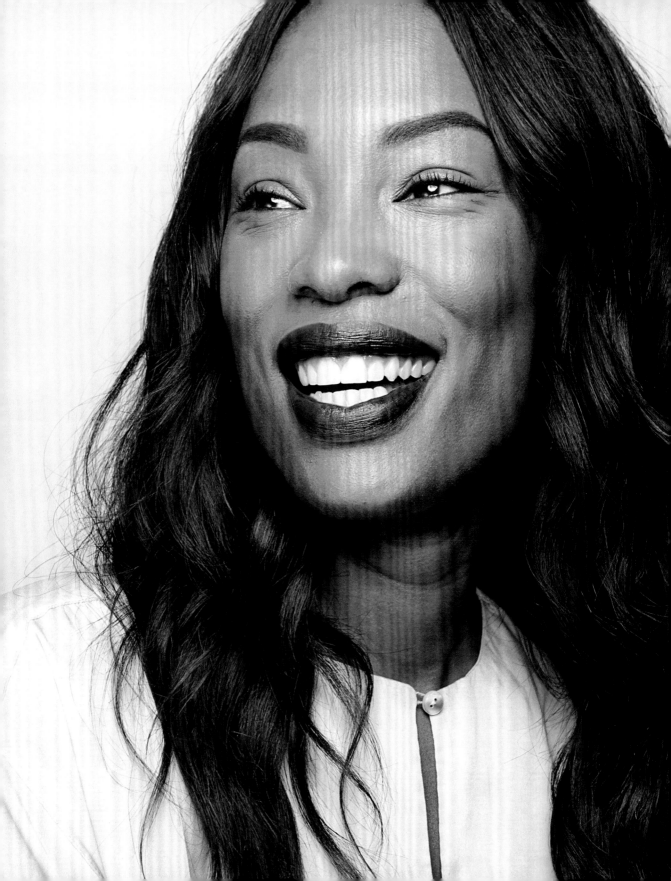

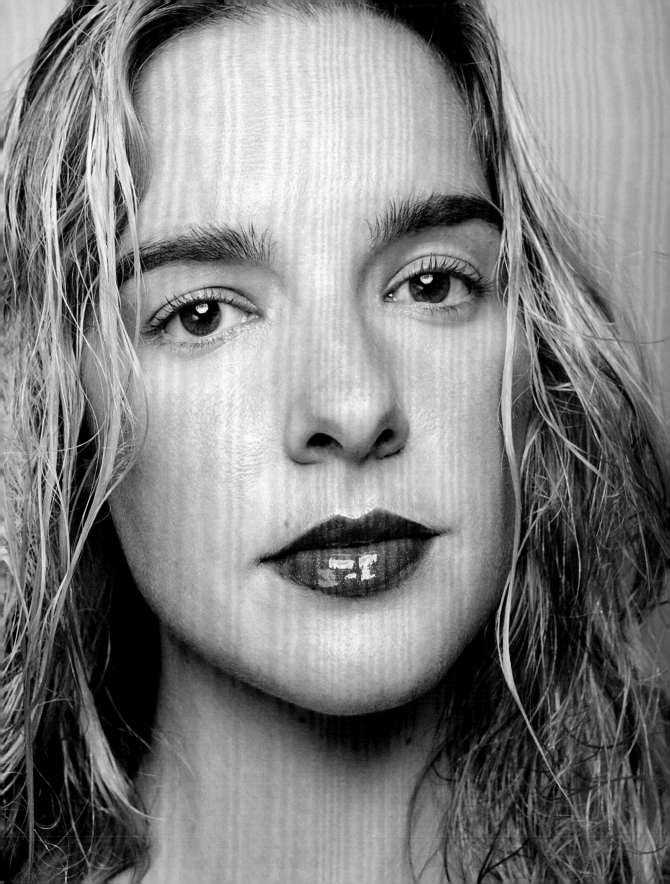

High shine gloss

Ahh lip gloss, one of the favourite and most annoying make-up products ever! People love gloss because it makes your lips look hydrated and gorgeous. But it's painful to wear because everything sticks to it. Don't even bother wearing it when there's a threat of high wind on the weather channel! And if you're going on a date then stick to lip balm! Ok, I may be being slightly dramatic. Things have changed and there are tons of non-stick glosses out there. But, let's be honest, the best glosses for that real 'wet look' are still the super-sticky ones. I use one in this look, but can you blame me?! Look how good it looks! Here's how to make the most of a glossy lip, sticky or not.

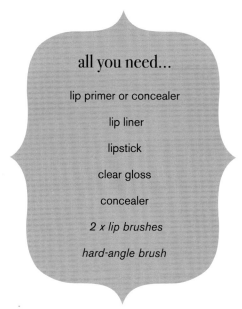

all you need...

lip primer or concealer

lip liner

lipstick

clear gloss

concealer

2 x lip brushes

hard-angle brush

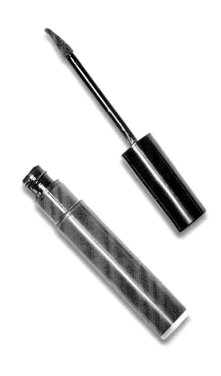

Keep base and eyes simple for this look – it's all about the lips after all. Use a touch of the same lips product on cheeks to match the lips and embrace the gorgeousness!

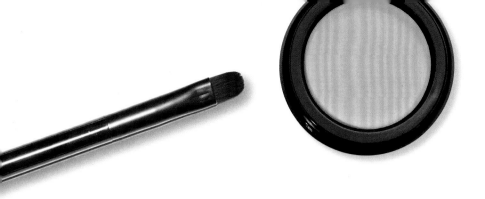

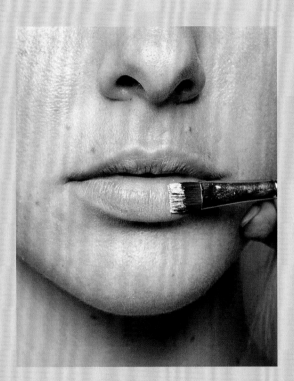

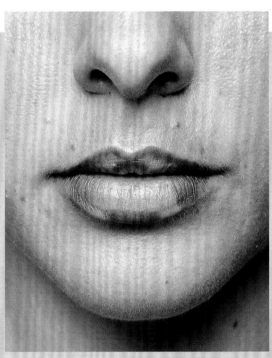

step 2 Line your lips with the bright lip liner. (You don't have to do this, but it will give you a more defined lip look. For a full guide on this see pages 120–123.)

step 1 Prime the lips with a lip primer or with concealer. Apply either product all over the lips with a lip brush. This will help to bring out the colour of your lipstick, as well as help to keep it in place.

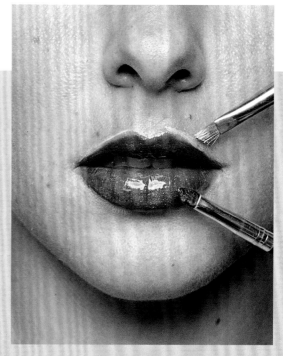

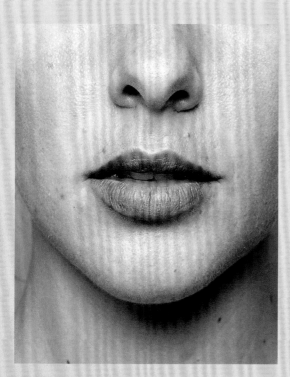

step 3 Fill in your lips with the lipstick. I like to use a lip brush for this, particularly if I've lined the lips. Remember a high shine lip works in any colour you like so be daring.

step 4 Now for the gloss. Either go for a clear gloss or one to match your lipstick and liner. Apply this all over the lip, starting from the centre and blending outwards. Glosses, especially the REALLY shiny ones, can be quite gloopy. So starting in the centre means you can spread out the excess. Again, I like to use a lip brush for precision. This also means I won't turn the lip gloss applicator (especially on a clear gloss) the colour of my lipstick! Finish by concealing around the edge of the lips using a hard-angle brush to sharpen the look.

Now stand really still, don't let any stray hairs cross your lips, oh and definitely don't eat a doughnut – the sugar will stick like glue! P.S. You look amazing so it's all worth it!

Highlighted lips

I've included this technique in the book, as whenever I do this look on myself, people always ask me what I've done differently to my lips as they love the look. Well it's pretty straightforward and it's a touch of highlighter that is key!

all you need...

lip primer

lipstick

lip liner (optional)

highlighter

clear gloss

2 x lip brushes

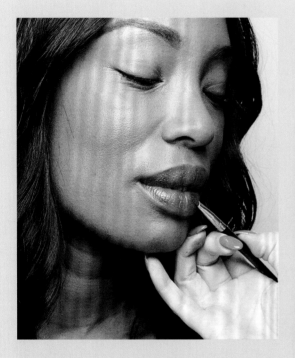

step 1 Apply your lipstick. (There are loads of tips on how to do this properly on pages 120–123.)

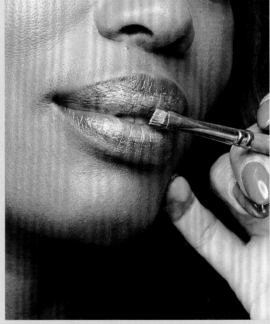

step 2 Take a highlighter. I prefer cream ones for this technique. Tone-wise, I find that highlighters with a gold or pink undertone work best too. Pat the highlighter, using your finger or a brush, onto the centre of the lips. As with contouring, the highlight pushes forward that section of the lip, making your lips look fuller.

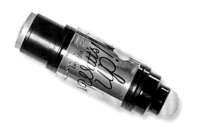

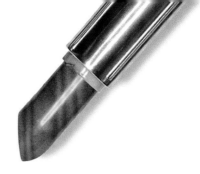

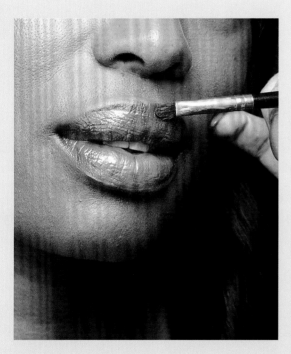

step 3 Go over the lips with a clear gloss. Blend from the centre out so that you don't remove the highlighter too far away from its original position.

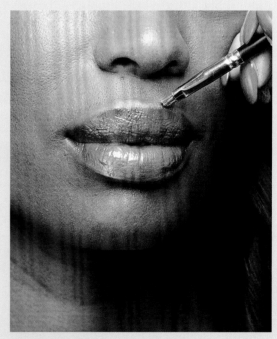

step 4 Highlight the cupid's bow of the lip for an extra glow and there you have it, bright, party-ready, highlighted lips!

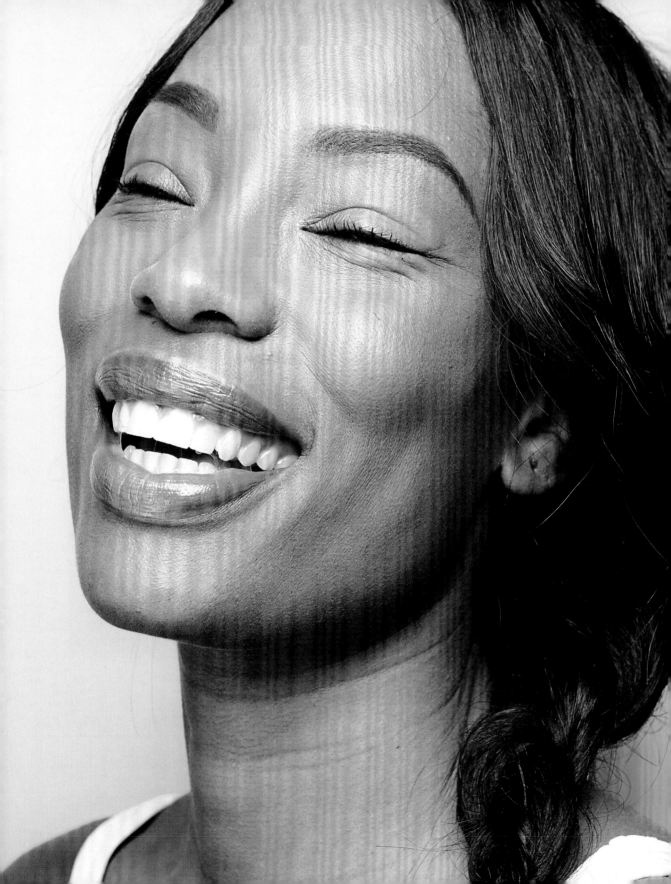

Highlighting isn't just for pink and red lips – look how amazing it looks on purple!

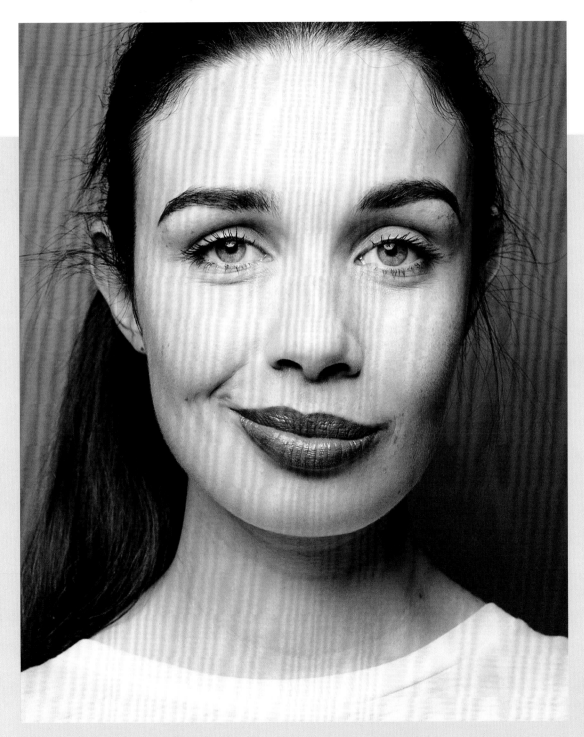

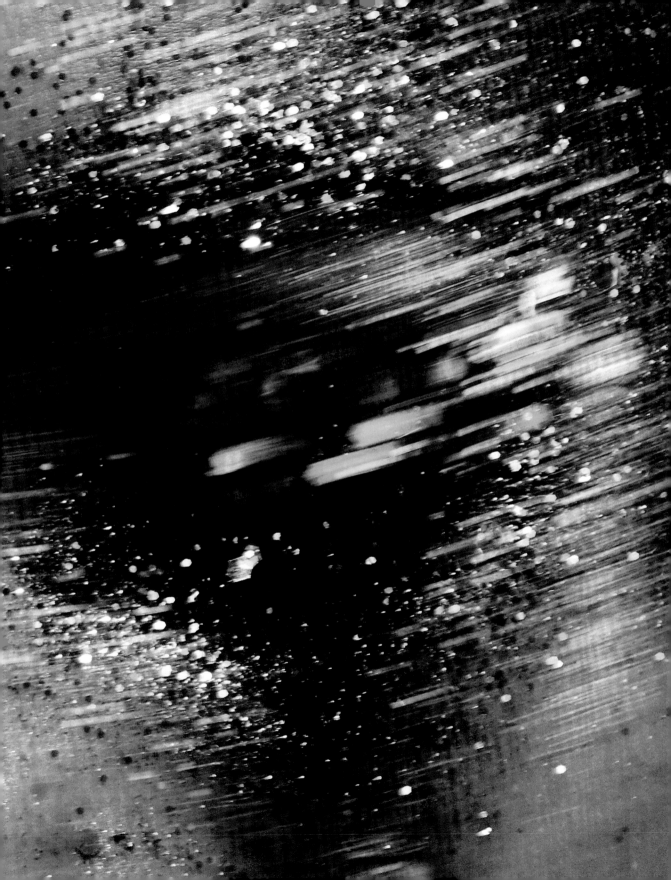

Looks to dazzle

Never let anyone dull your sparkle!

One day, my cat Kimmy rolled in a pile of glitter that I'd split on my kitchen floor. She's never looked more beautiful and I'm pretty sure she loved it as she began strutting around like some sort of supermodel! Ha! I love glitter. My husband does not love glitter quite as much. Mainly because it's all over our house and going into an important meeting, accidently sparkling like a galaxy of stars is probably not ideal, for him anyway! My friend Neil has a minor phobia of glitter. I'm the most unsympathetic friend he has, as you can imagine! I once baked him a glittery birthday cake, much to his horror and my delight. So yes, glitter, sequins, sparkly things, I love them! I collect vintage ball gowns (only the sparkly ones of course) and even my sun cream has glitter in it (it's Ultrasun Glimmer in case you wondered).

So this section of the book makes me very happy. From a touch of glitter to a glittery lip. A bit of sparkle never harmed anyone.

A little sparkle

Adding even a touch of glitter to your make-up can transform your look. And glitter isn't just for teenagers, anyone can wear it. If you're older, then a sheer glitter over a nude lid can look wonderful. As does a slick of glitter over an eyeliner flick (see page 93). In fact, there are loads of sophisticated glitter products out there, meaning you can choose to sparkle as little or as much as you like. For this look, I add a small amount of glitter into the corner of the eyes. This is perfect for a night out, the festive season, or for a Tuesday at work when you want to brighten up the office!

all you need...

loose eye glitter

clear gloss or Vaseline

medium pencil brush

lip brush

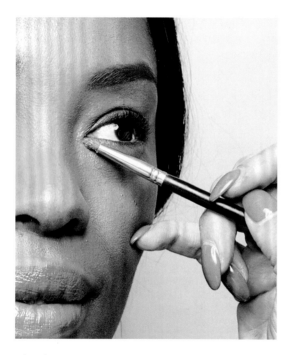

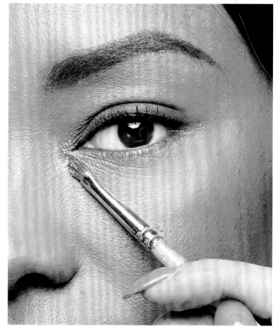

step 1 Pick your glitter. Remember to always use a glitter that is made for use near the eyes. Don't use a craft glitter as these are very sharp and can damage your eyes. Take a medium pencil brush, a clear gloss or Vaseline and dot this wherever you would like the glitter to sit. For this look I dot it in the corner of the eye where it will catch the light and make your eyes shine.

step 2 Add the loose eye glitter. I love to use a lip brush to do this as I find it's less messy and more precise.

And that's it! You are now more sparkly than you were about 30 seconds ago, yay!

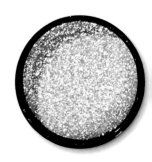

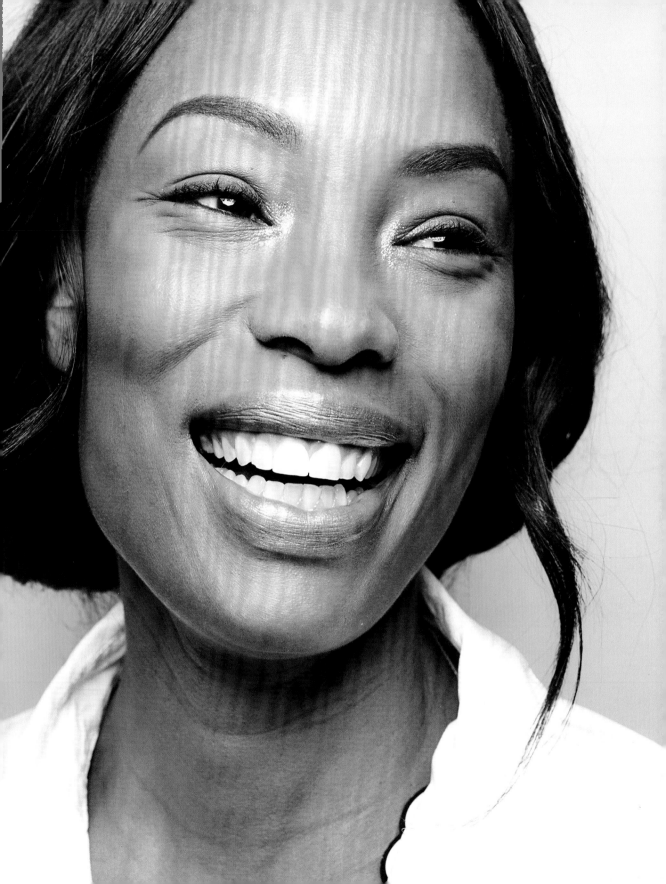

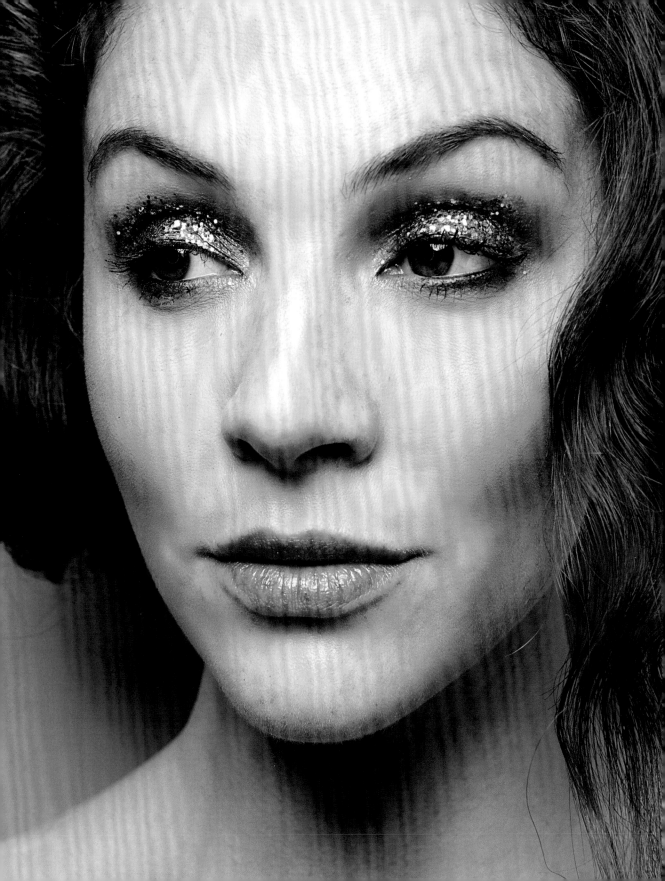

A touch more sparkle

A full-on glittery eye is always a winner. And you can add glitter to any eye look. Here, I glitter up the Bronze Shadow (see pages 106–109) with glitter shades that work well with the bronze: one loose glitter in gold and one glitter eyeshadow in bronze.

all you need...

loose face powder

loose eye glitter

glitter eyeshadow

clear gloss or Vaseline

blending sponge

flat eyeshadow brush

blusher brush

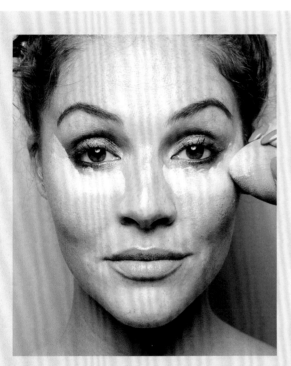

step 1 Create your chosen eye look. Do your brows and base too. Then pat a loose face powder under the eyes with a sponge. This will catch any of the glitter that falls beneath. (We will sweep this away at the end so that you don't have to redo your concealer or foundation.)

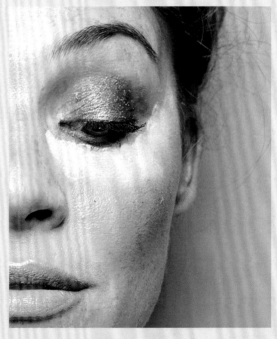

step 2 Pat the glitter eyeshadow over the eye look, focusing on the centre of the eye. Use a flat eyeshadow brush as this will make sure the glitter sits well on the eye. This will act as a good base for the loose eye glitter.

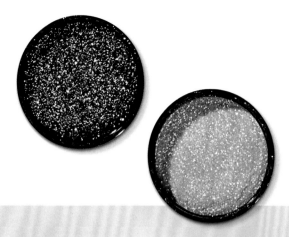

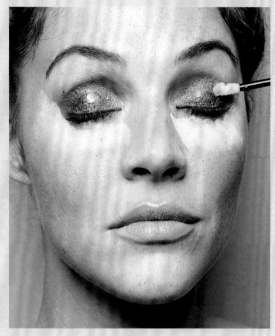

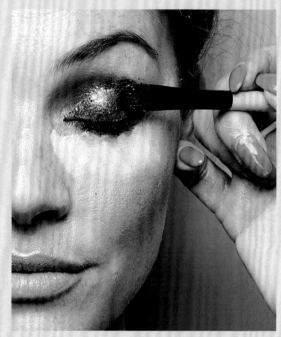

step 3 Pat a small amount of clear gloss or Vaseline over the lid.

step 4 Press the loose eye glitter over the top of the gloss using a fluffy eyeshadow brush and layer until you have enough shine.

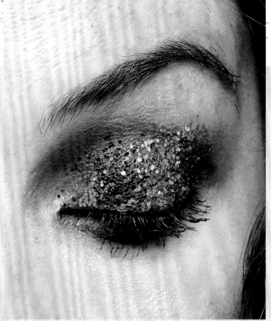

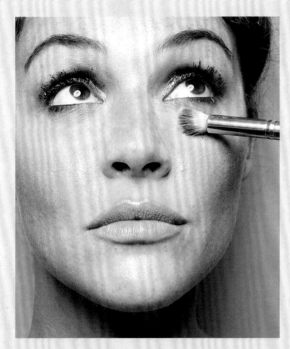

step 5 Sweep away the loose face powder from underneath your eyes with a blusher brush to get rid of any excess glitter that has fallen onto the cheeks. (If you're wearing a black top, cover it with something. Glitter falling on your top is nice, powder falling on it? Not so much!)

Top tip

If you find there is still glitter on your face, use a small amount of masking tape to remove it. (Do not use Sellotape as this will remove your make-up!)

Wedding make-up dos and don'ts

It's the best day of your life so you want to look amazing. Don't do what I did and do your wedding make up in 3 minutes and 56 seconds (long story)! Follow my dos and don'ts for a stress-free day. Oh, and congratulations!!!

The dos

DO Have a make-up trial. Have it no sooner than 5 weeks before the big day. If you have your trial in January but the wedding is in July, your skin tone will be completely different. So 3–5 weeks before is ideal. If you're doing your own make-up, practise a few times first.

DO Wear a loose, white T-shirt to your make-up trial (or a colour t-shirt nearest to the colour of your dress) This way you can see how the make up looks against the colour. (Oh, and on the wedding day, wear a loose t-shirt so that you don't ruin your hair and make-up when you go to put on your dress.)

DO Step into natural light after your make-up trial. Take pictures with and without a flash. If your make-up looks great in natural light, it will look great anywhere.

DO Prepare. By this I mean, if you're going to have a fake tan, individual lashes or body waxing, don't have them for the first time the day before the wedding. Trial them months before to make sure you like the look.

DO Have a massage the day before the wedding. This will relax you and let you enjoy the big day even more.

DO follow this order on the actual day. If you're having your hair set in rollers, make sure you have this done first. This will give it longer to set while you are having your make-up done, meaning it will last longer throughout the day. Also, make sure the mother of the bride has

her hair and make-up done as soon as possible, if not first. She'll want to be running around organizing things, and on more than one occasion, I've seen the M. O. B. run out of time. So get her sorted first, then she can help you with any errands, while still feeling gorgeous and glam.

DO Use primer! This is vital for your skin and eyes as it will lock in your make-up and make it last much longer.

DO Use a foundation that you know and love. Take it with you to your trial. You want your skin to look the way you like it.

DO Give your bridesmaids your lipstick, powder and blusher. These are the three products that might need touching up throughout the day.

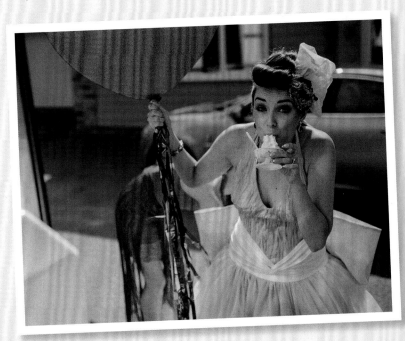

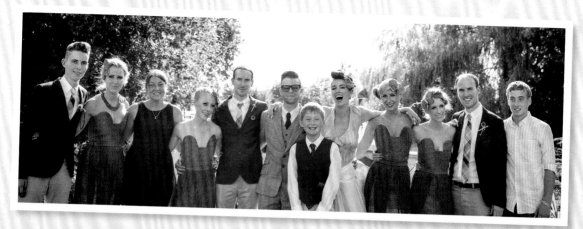

The don'ts

DON'T Wear a bra or socks when you're getting ready! The marks are so hard to get rid of (imagine bra strap marks with a strapless dress)!

DON'T Change your skincare routine too close to the big day. This can cause breakouts and NOBODY wants that!

DON'T Let your make-up artist hijack your big day. Go to the trial with an idea of what you want. Take pictures with you and stick to it.

DON'T Go too heavy with your make-up. You want to enhance your natural beauty and look like the best version of yourself. You don't want to look like you're wearing a mask. Your other half may not recognize you when you reach the bottom of the aisle if you cake your make-up on!

DON'T Go for dark, black or grey eye make-up (unless that's your thing). Go for bronzes and defined eyes instead. The Bronze Shadow on pages 106–109 is perfect bridal make-up.

DON'T Rush! Your bridal make-up can take 45–90 minutes so make sure you plan it into the schedule (unlike me).

DON'T Follow trends. Although those eyeliner dots under the eyes may seem cool now, you will want to look through your wedding photos forever with admiration, without thinking, 'why did I do that?'

DON'T Wear too much blusher. You'll be so excited, nervous and happy that you'll have a lot of natural colour in your cheeks, so avoid red and deep pink blushers.

DON'T Forget your brows! Have them waxed and tinted a week before the wedding. They frame your face and a groomed brow makes such a difference in photos.

DON'T Wear sticky lip gloss! Think about it, first kiss. HUGE photo opportunity. Sticking to your new husband or wife is not ideal! Neither is the stringy lip gloss between the two of you scenario – eurgh!

DON'T Forget to have a glass of Champagne. It's your special day, relax and enjoy every second!

Top tip

For the evening part of the wedding, pat a touch of glitter into the centre of the eye, and add a deeper lipstick. It's your biggest party EVER! So why not glam it up?

Glitter lips

Ok, so this is the most fabulous, unwearable make-up look in the entire book! But I challenge each and every one of you to give it a go as you will feel, and look, just wonderful! (Just remember to drink through a straw and try not to kiss anyone – everyone will know if you do!) I first tried a glitter lip when I was 14 years old. I was going to the annual school disco and got my hands on some glitter from my mum's craft box. I literally sprinkled some glitter onto a plate, chucked on some lip gloss and stuck my lips into it! I swallowed nearly as much glitter as I had on my lips, but it looked amazing and received many compliments that night! Since then, I've discovered cleaner and less dangerous ways to apply glitter to my lips! Recently legendary make-up artist, Pat Mcgrath, has produced glitter lip kits! The glitter is super-fine and sparkly so it's perfect for the lips. However, it's also pretty hard to get your hands on, so a clear gloss and a fine glitter from any make-up brand will do just fine.

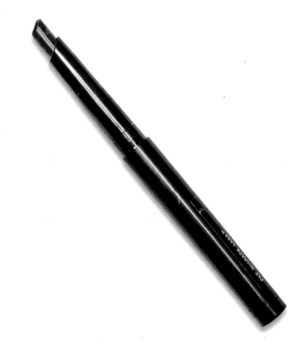

all you need...

lip exfoliator

concealer

lip primer

lip liner

lipstick

clear gloss

fine glitter

tissue

lip brush

pencil brush

tissue or masking tape

thin lip brush

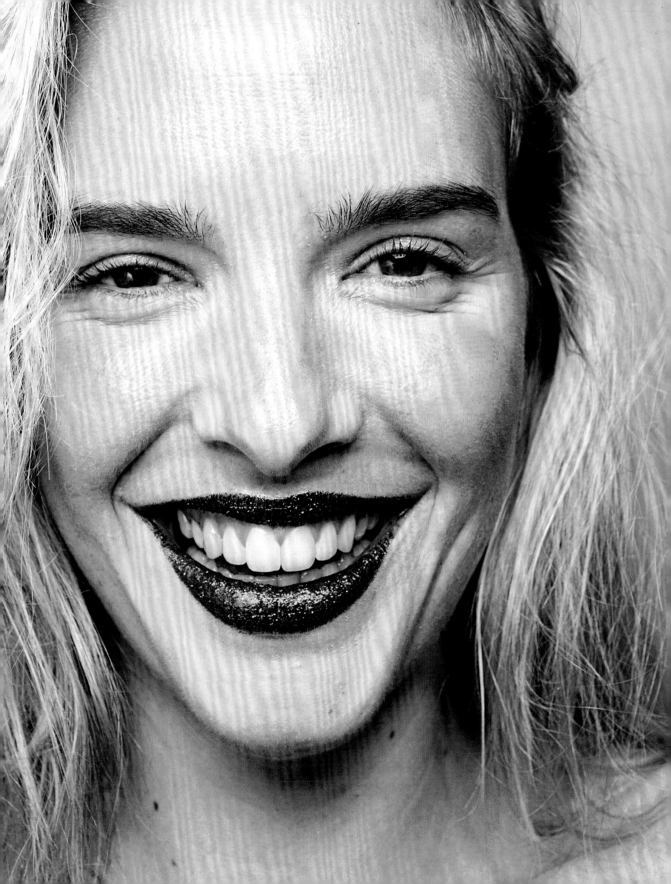

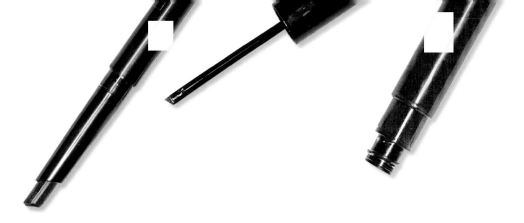

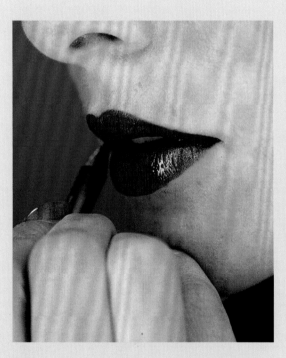

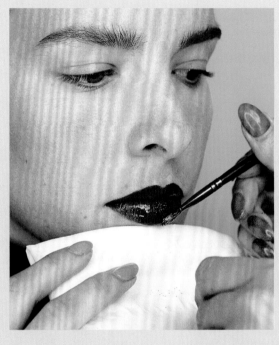

step 1 Start by creating the perfect red lip (see pages 120–123). Obviously, if you're going for a different coloured glitter, match your lipstick to that. Then add a clear gloss over the top.

step 2 Hold a piece of tissue (or gently masking tape it in place) underneath your lip line, covering your chin. Fine glitter is the hardest to remove so this trick will save you loads of time and effort. Next, take a thin lip brush and start to press the glitter into the lip, working from the centre outwards. It's important that you gently press it on to ensure that it sticks.

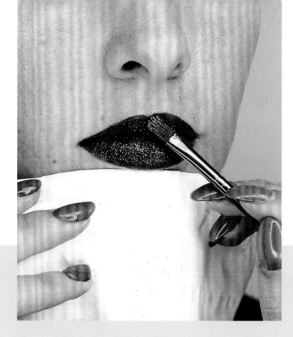

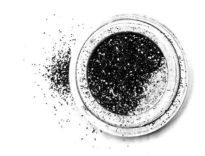

step 3 Take your time! Don't try to add too much at once. This is a labour of love, but oh, so worth it! If you get any excess glitter outside of the lip line. Just remove it with a tiny bit of masking tape.

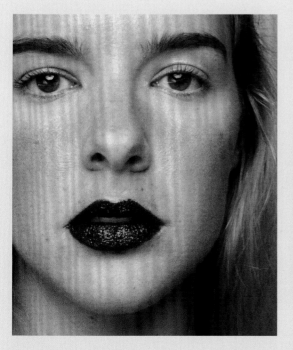

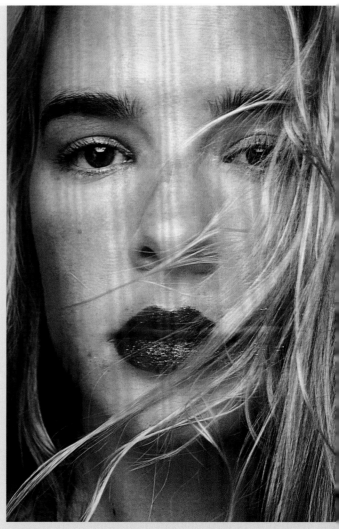

Glitter lip of joy complete. Now, no kissing, eating, licking your lips or drinking without a straw.

Halloween

I love Halloween! It's the perfect time to get really creative with make-up. I also LOVE seeing what other make-up artists create at this time of the year. There's so much cool stuff out there! I regularly publish 'Halloween Week' online on my YouTube channel, creating a whole week's worth of Halloween make-up tutorials. Here are a few of my faves.

I have given you some hints and tips for creating these looks below but you can see the full tutorials for each of these looks at www.youtube.com/lisapotterdixon. Subscribe as I post two videos a week. Enjoy!

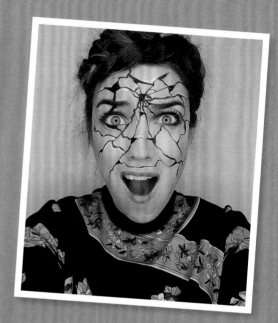

✱ My favourite face paints are by Snazaroo. These are what my mum used to use on me when I was little. They are the best and tend to stay in place the longest.

✱ You can buy zips from most party shops. If not, just buy a zip from a fabric shop and trim away the edges, leaving just the metal zip.

✱ Coloured contact lenses are amazing for finishing your Halloween looks. Just make sure you try them out before the big day as they may irritate the eyes and you don't want your Halloween make-up to turn into an actual nightmare.

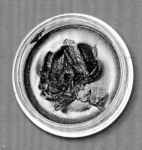

✱ I have a full-on fancy dress box with wigs and outfits galore! If you don't have access to fancy dress, don't worry. Apart from the facepaint, the quickest way to transform your look is with a wig. Amazon has lots of different options available for relatively low cost!

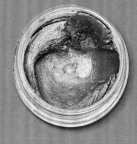

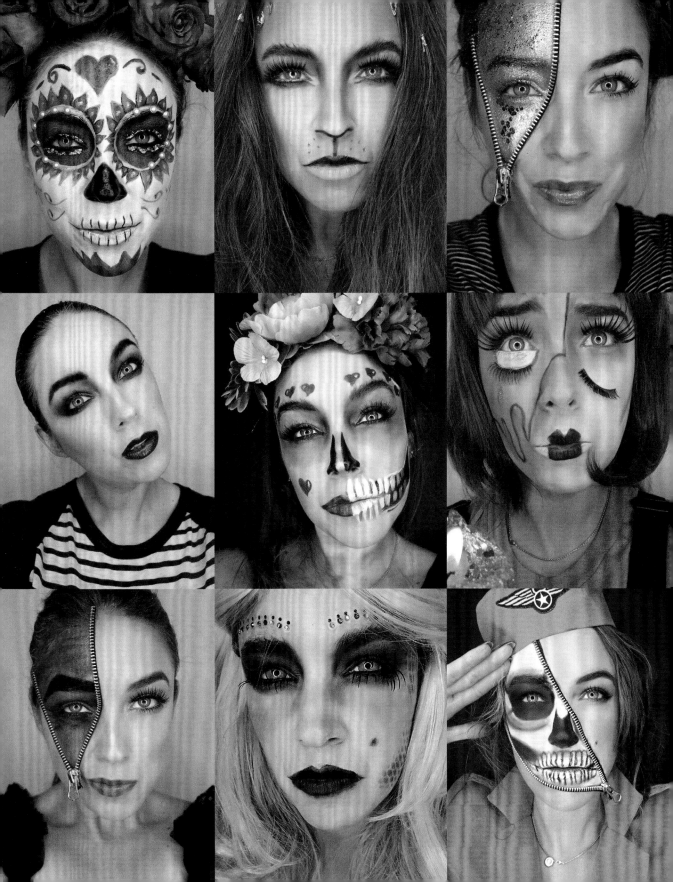

Extreme glitter

I LOVE this look! Whether you're going to a festival, a Christmas party or you just fancy adding some extra sparkle to your Saturday night, I dare you to give this a go.

all you need...

metallic cream eyeshadow

glitter gel eye liner

foil sequins

mascara

eyeshadow brush

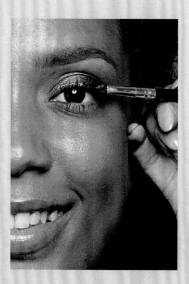

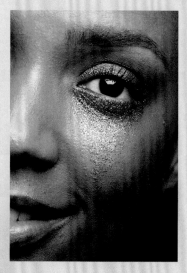

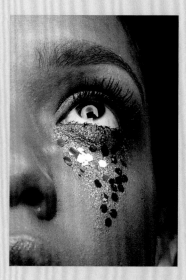

step 1 Start by applying a metallic cream eyeshadow of your choice all over your eyelid up into the socket.

step 2 Use a glittery gel eye liner to draw a solid triangle under your eye. Again, any colour is good – it's a party, people! There are no rules. Repeat this under the other eye if you like, or just keep it to one. Add layers of black mascara (see page 82).

step 3 While the liner is still wet, scatter some foil sequins over the triangle(s) to add extra sparkle.

You are now, officially, a sparkly unicorn of joy! You're welcome.

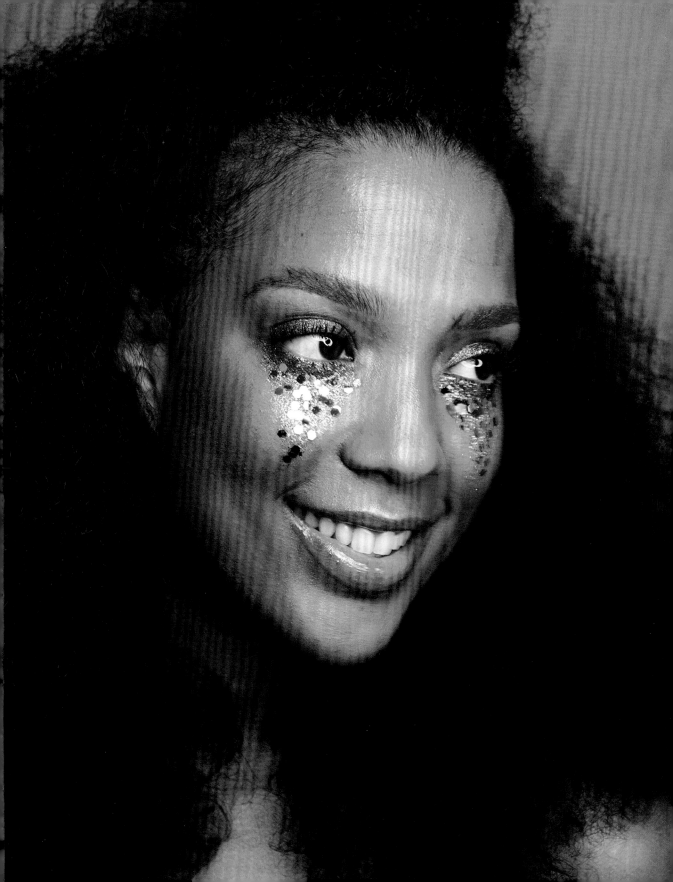

All you need... (in detail)

32 Benefit: lemonaid colour corrector; hello flawless oxygen wow! *I'm so money (honey)*; boi-ing *02*; the POREfessional agent zero shine.

34–35 Sephora: Sephora + PANTONE UNIVERSE Correct + Conceal Palette. Benefit: hello flawless! oxygen wow *show me the money (honey)*; stay don't stray *light/medium*; the POREfessional: agent zero shine; rollerlash mascara *black*; high brow glow; hoola; precisley my brow pencil *02 – light*; dandelion; they're real! double the lip *lusty rose*. Marc Jacobs: Style Eye-con *No. 7 Plush Eyeshadow The Dreamer 212*.

40–41 and 50–51 Same as page 32 plus Benefit: brow-vo conditioning primer; precisley my brow pencil *04 – medium*; gimme brow *03 – medium*.

42 Benefit: the POREfessional; hello flawless oxygen wow! *I'm all the rage (beige)*; stay don't stray *light/medium*; boi-ing *02*; gimme brow *05 – deep*; hoola. Illamasqua: Beyond Highlighter.

43 Benefit: precisely, my brow pencil *02 – light*; gimme brow *01 – light*; ready, set, BROW!

44–45 Same as pages 74–75 plus Benefit: gimme brow *05 – deep*.

46–49 Benefit: hello flawless oxygen wow! *I'm so money (honey)*; hello flawless oxygen wow! *I'm all the rage (beige)*; stay don't stray *light/medium*; hoola; ka-brow *04 – medium*.

52–53 Benefit: sunbeam; hello flawless oxygen wow! *I'm so money (honey)*; stay don't stray *light/medium*; boi-ing *02*; hoola; ka-brow *05 – deep*; gimme brow *05 – deep*.

58 Make Up For Ever: HD Foundation *175 – R510 Coffee*. Nars: Sheer Glow Foundation *New Orleans*. Amazing Cosmetics: Amazing Concealer *Medium Beige*. Mary Kay: Facial Highlighting Pen *Shade 4*. AJ Crimson Beauty: Universal Finishing Powder *Bamboo*. Benefit: precisely, my brow pencil *06 – deep*; gimme brow *05 – deep*. Mac: Powder Blush *Plum Foolery*. Danessa Myricks: Enlight Halo Powder *Heat*.

66–69 Benefit: hello flawless! oxygen wow *show me the money (honey)*; stay don't stray *light/medium*; hoola; rockateur; ka-BROW! *04 – medium*; precisely, my brow pencil *05 – deep*; rollerlash mascara *black*. Anastasia Beverly Hills: The Original Contour Kit. Rodial: Instaglam Compact Deluxe Illuminating Powder. YSL: Rouge Pur Couture Satin Radiance Lipstick *51 Corail Urbain*.

70 Same as page 43 plus Benefit: the POREfessional, hello flawless! oxygen wow *show me the money (honey)*; fakeup *01 – light*; hoola; hervana. Nars: Velvet Matte Lip Pencil *Damned*.

72–73 Benefit: hello flawless oxygen wow! *I'm pure for sure (ivory)*; dew the hoola liquid bronzer; precisley my brow pencil *05 – deep*;

hoola; they're real! mascara *black*. Danessa Myricks: Enlight Attraction. Crown Brush: Crystal Lip Gloss.

74–75 Benefit: the POREfessional; hello flawless oxygen wow! *I'm so money (honey)*; hello flawless oxygen wow! *cheers to me (Champagne)*; brow zings *04 – medium*; precisely my brow pencil *05 – deep*.

86–88 Same as pages 46–49 plus Benefit: they're real! push-up liner *black*; they're real! mascara *black*; boi-ing *02*; Benetint.

90–93 Same as pages 74–75 plus Benefit: rollerlash mascara *black*. Make Up For Ever: Kohl Liner *8k*. Barry M: Dazzle Dust *Petrol Black*.

94–96 Benefit: goof proof pencil *06 – deep*; ready, set, BROW; they're real! mascara *blue*. Make Up For Ever: HD Foundation *caramel*; Aqua Eye Pencil *M26*. Amazing Cosmetics: Concealer *medium beige*.

97 Same as pages 52–53 plus Benefit: they're real mascara *blue*; benetint. Nars: Velvet Shadow Stick *Glenan*.

98–99 Same as page 32 plus Benefit: rollerlash mascara *black*; Make Up For Ever: Artist Shadow Palette *01*.

100–103 Benefit: hello flawless! oxygen wow *show me the money (honey)*; stay don't stray *light/medium*; hoola; rockateur; ka-

BROW! *04 – medium*; precisely, my brow pencil *05 – deep*; they're real! mascara *black*; benetint; they're real: double the lip *juicy berry*. Make Up For Ever: Artist Shadow Palette *01*. Illamasqua: Precision Gel Liner *Infinity*.

104–105 Same as pages 52–53 plus Benefit: they're real mascara *black*; they're real double the lip *nude scandal*. Nars: Velvet Shadow Stick *Sukhothai*; Velvet Matte Lip Pencil *Damned*. Estee Lauder: Edit 02 *Aqua Nova*. Marc Jacobs: Black Gel Crayon. Revlon: Ultra HD 500 Lip Gloss *Garnet*.

105 (top left) Same as page 42 plus Benefit: bad gal mascara *black*; they're real! mascara *black*. Urban Decay: Eyeshadow *Danger*.

106–109 Benefit: the POREfessional; hello flawless! oxygen wow *I'm so money (honey)*; sun beam; stay don't stray *light/ medium*; boi-ing *02*; hoola; goof proof eyebrow pencil *03 – medium*; gimme brow *03 – medium*; ready, set, BROW! clear brow gel; bad gal eyeliner *black*; they're real! mascara *black*. Marc Jacobs Style Eye-con *No. 7 Plush Eyeshadow The Dreamer 212*.

110–113 Same as pages 66–69 plus Benefit: they're real! mascara *black*; they're real push-up liner *black*. Marc Jacobs Style Eye-con *No. 7 Plush Eyeshadow The Dreamer 212*. Danessa Myricks: Elevation Lashes Uplift *02*.

120–123 Same as pages 72–73 plus Make Up For Ever: Aqua Lip *08C Red*; Artist Rouge Crème *C404 Passion Red*. Benefit: boi-ing *01*.

124–125 Same as pages 106–109 plus Benefit: stay don't stray *light/ medium*. Mac: Lip Pencil *Subculture*. Make Up For Ever: Artist Rouge Cream Lipstick *C104 Praline Beige*.

126–127 YSL: Rouge Pur Couture Satin Radiance Lipstick *Blond Ingenu*. Benefit: hello flawless oxygen wow! *I'm pure for sure (ivory)*; hello flawless oxygen wow! *I'm all money (honey)*; rollerlash mascara *black*; ready, set, BROW.

128–129 Same as page 58 plus GLAMGLOW Poutmud Wet Lip Balm Treatment. Pat McGrath Labs: Lust 004 Kits *Bloodwine*.

130–133 Same as pages 52–53 plus Benefit: boi-ing *02*. Make Up For Ever: Lip Liner *17c Bright Orange*; Artist Rouge Cream *C304 Orange*. Crown Brush: Crystal Lip Gloss.

134–136 Same as page 58 plus YSL: Rouge Pur Couture Satin Radiance Lipstick *07 Le Fuschia*. Benefit: watt's up; ultra plush lip gloss *icebreaker*.

137 Same as pages 72–73 plus Too Faced: Melted Liquified Long Wear Lipstick *Melted Violet*.

140–141 Same as page 58 plus Vaseline. In Your Dreams: Fine Glitter *Iridescent Angel*.

142–145 Same as pages 106–109 plus Charlotte Tilbury: Luxury Palette *The Dolce Vita*. In Your Dreams: Chunky Angelic Glitter *Gold Lileth*.

148–151 Same as pages 52–53 plus Pat Mcgrath: Lust 004 Kit *Vermillion Venom*.

154–155 Same as pages 94–96 plus Make Up For Ever: Aqua Cream *19 Purple*; Extra Large Size Glitter. Urban Decay: Glitter Eye Liner *Heavy Metal*. In Your Dreams: Blue Frosted Fairy Chunky Glitter.

Essential tools

beautyblender® Classic
Favourite brushes:
Crown Brush *www.crownbrush. co.uk*
Make Up For Ever *www.makeupforever.com*
Real Techniques *www.realtechniques.com*
Wayne Goss *www.gossmakeup.com*
Zoeva *www.zoevacosmetics.com*

Resources

AJ Crimson Beauty
www.ajcrimson.com

Amazing Cosmetics
www.amazingcosmetics.com

Anastasia Beverly Hills
www.anastasiabeverlyhills.com

ARDELL
www.ardelllashes.com

Balance Me
www.balanceme.co.uk

Barry M
www.barrym.com

beautyblender®
www.beautyblender.com

Benefit Cosmetics
www.benefitcosmetics.co.uk
www.benefitcosmetics.com

Boots
www.boots.com

Cetaphil
www.cetaphil.com

Chanel
www.chanel.com

Charlotte Tilbury
www.charlottetilbury.com

LA MER
www.cremedelamer.com

Crown Brush
www.crownbrush.co.uk

Danessa Myricks Beauty
www.danessamyricks
beauty.com

DUO®
www.duoadhesives.com

E45
www.e45.co.uk

ELEMIS®
www.elemis.com

Estée Edit
www.esteelauder.com

EVE LOM
www.evelom.com

Fleur de Force by Eylure
www.eylure.com/fleur-de-force

Fresh Cosmetics
www.fresh.com

GLAMGLOW
www.glamglow.com

Goldfaden MD
www.goldfadenmd.com

Illamasqua
www.illamasqua.com

In Your Dreams
www.inyour-dreams.com

Lisa Potter-Dixon
www.lisapotterdixon.com
www.youtube.com/lisapotterdixon
@Lisa_Benefit

Lucas' Papaw Remedies
www.lucaspapaw.com.au

MAC Cosmetics
www.maccosmetics.com

Make Up For Ever
www.makeupforever.com

Marc Jacobs Beauty
www.marcjacobsbeauty.com

Mary Kay
www.marykay.com

Murad
www.murad.com

NARS Cosmetics
www.narscosmetics.com

Nip+Fab
www.nipandfab.com

Nivea
www.nivea.co.uk
www.niveausa.com

Onira Organics Haircare
www.oniraorganics.com

OPI Products Inc.
www.opi.com

Pat McGrath Labs
www.patmcgrath.com

Perricone MD®
www.perriconemd.com

Rodial
www.rodial.com

Sanctuary Spa
www.sanctuary.com

Sephora
www.sephora.com

Too Faced
www.toofaced.com

Tweezerman®
www.tweezerman.com

Urban Decay
www.urbandecay.com

Vaseline
www.vaseline.co.uk
www.vaseline.us

Vita Coco®
www.vitacoco.com

YSL Beauty
www.yslbeauty.co.uk
www.yslbeautyus.com

Index

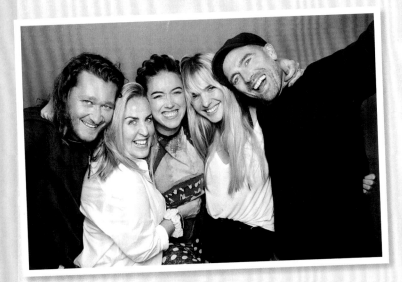

Acknowledgments

Wow, book number two! I can't quite believe it. What a labour of love it has been! I've loved every minute of it, but there's definitely been a lot of people who have kept me going through this journey…

Firstly, thank you to everyone who has bought this book and who continues to follow my journey, for all your support. You guys are the absolute best!

To my incredible husband, Theo. The only one who has really seen the late nights, early mornings, tears and passion that have gone into this book. Thank you for encouraging me and always keeping me positive. I couldn't do what I do without you. I love you, I love you, I love you. #AimEverHigher.

Snoopy and Kimmy, rolling in all the glitter and stamping mud all over the book as I'm trying to write it is never ideal, but the constant cuddles make up for it! Thanks for being the best pup and kitty cat in the land!

To my friends, you know who you are. Thank you for the cuddles, the chats and the coffee when I've needed a break. You continue to fill my life with laughter and happiness. A special, HUGE thank you to Rosie, Emzie, Caz, Clare, Ky, Dano, Dom, Andy, Franny, Lex, Laura, Soph, Dawny, Lucy, Kate, Emi, Jenna and Tana, for listening, laughing and advising me whatever the hour.

To my family, thank you for always believing in me and inspiring me. I love you all.

To my awesome book team, Rhys (snaps) and Matt (hair). You guys have made this experience so fun and pretty damn epic! I truly couldn't have done it without you both (and the Minapples). I'm so grateful to have met two such creative, crazy guys and can't wait to see what our next project entails. But, more importantly, can't wait to see which Snapchat filter Matt rocks next! Love you both.

To the greatest team in the game, Lauren and Laurretta. Thank you for your constant support, jokes, laughter, meditation and dance moves. I'm so lucky to have a team that always keep the (Prosecco) glass half full! Love you both, you know that.

To my fab publishers, Ryland Peters & Small. Thank you for wanting to work with me again and for letting me roll with all my crazy ideas. BIG thanks to Steph, Barbara, Leslie, Julia and Cindy for pushing me and believing in me always. I'm very proud of what we have achieved.

To my Benefit family, thank you for just being the best! Special thanks to Gail, Ian, Andrea and Sarah for always supporting me 100 per cent. I'm forever grateful.

To all the beautiful ladies who have modelled for me in this book, you made my job easy. Thanks for going with the (very fast) flow. You make this book very special.

All hail my nails! To my friend, Michael Do, the only person allowed to go near my nails! Thank you for keeping them on point for the whole book. You the best. @Michaeldo92.

Sally, thank you for the gorgeous illustrations once again. I so appreciate you squeezing them into your busy schedule and I am very proud of all you are achieving. @sally_faye.

Soph and Sonia, thanks so much for your wonderful kind words. Your support throughout my career has been so important to me. You are two incredible women. Thank you.

To everyone in the industry who continues to believe in me and take a chance on me. Thank you.

To all my fellow make-up artists how lucky are we to get to do what we love?! Thank you for inspiring me with all your beautiful creations.

To all the aspiring make-up artists out there, follow your dreams, work hard and never give up.

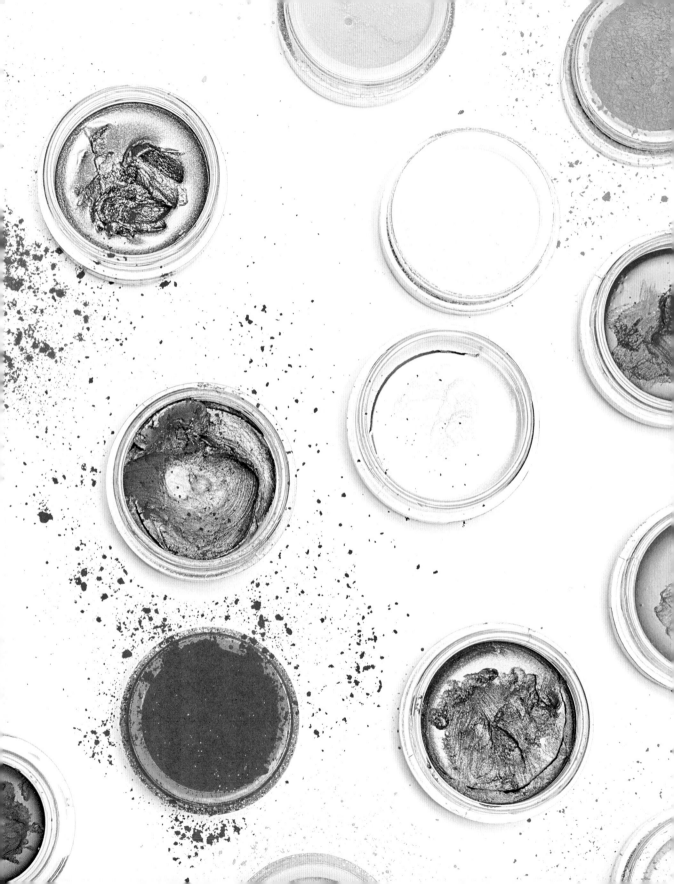